100 CASES
in Orthopaedics and Rheumatology

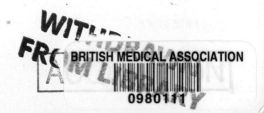

100 CASES
in Orthopaedics and Rheumatology

Parminder J. Singh MBBS MRCS FRCS(Tr&Orth) MS
Consultant Orthopaedic & Trauma Surgeon and Senior Lecturer, Maroondah Hospital,
Monash and Deakin University, Melbourne, Australia

Catherine Swales MRCP PhD
Arthritis Research UK Clinical Research Fellow and Clinical Lecturer in
Rheumatology, Nuffield Orthopaedic Centre, Oxford, UK

100 Cases Series Editor:
Professor P John Rees MD FRCP
Professor of Medical Education, King's College London School of Medicine at Guy's,
King's and St Thomas' Hospitals, London, UK

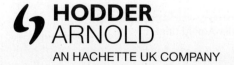
HODDER
ARNOLD
AN HACHETTE UK COMPANY

First published in Great Britain in 2012 by
Hodder Arnold, an imprint of Hodder Education, Hodder and Stoughton Ltd,
a division of Hachette UK
338 Euston Road, London NW1 3BH

http://www.hodderarnold.com

© 2012 Parminder J. Singh and Catherine Swales

British Library Cataloguing in Publication Data
A catalogue record for this book is available from the British Library

Library of Congress Cataloging-in-Publication Data
A catalog record for this book is available from the Library of Congress

ISBN-13 978-1-444-11794-3

1 2 3 4 5 6 7 8 9 10

Commissioning Editor:	Joanna Koster
Project Editor:	Jenny Wright
Production Controller:	Francesca Wardell
Cover Design:	Amina Dudhia
Index:	Lisa Footitt

Typeset in 10/12pt RotisSerif by Phoenix Photosetting, Chatham, Kent
Printed and bound in India

What do you think about this book? Or any other Hodder Arnold title?
Please visit our website: www.hodderarnold.com

CONTENTS

RHEUMATOLOGY

ACKNOWLEDGEMENTS

CS would like to thank colleagues in the Rheumatology, Radiology and Respiratory departments for their expertise, advice and invaluable contributions.

PJS: I would like to dedicate this book to my wife Rowena and children Kieran and Angelina Singh who have been as committed as I have in completing this book. Without their support and abundance of love none of this would be possible. I thank them enormously for their support. I would like to acknowledge my mother Gurbaksh Kaur for her lifetime support and love in making this all possible. I am very grateful for the opportunity to write this book and thank Professor Christopher Bulstrode in Oxford for this. Finally I would like to acknowledge two of my dearest and closest friends Richard and Lisa Field for their expert support and guidance throughout my professional life.

CASE 1: A PAINFUL KNEE IN A NEONATE

History

A young primigravida mother has become concerned about her newborn child. She is accompanied in the clinic by her aunt who recognized that something was not quite right but was not sure what to advise. The baby has general symptoms of fever, fatigue, irritability and malaise. There is no history of trauma.

Examination

Close inspection of the left leg reveals some localized oedema and erythema. On palpation the baby appears to have pain overlying the proximal tibia. Passive manipulation shows a full range of movement of the leg without any obvious indications of pain.

Investigations

Initial investigations show a markedly elevated C-reactive protein (CRP). Imaging studies of the knee show periosteal elevation of the proximal tibial metaphysis (Fig. 1.1).

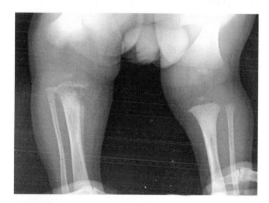

Figure 1.1

Questions

- What is the diagnosis?
- What are the radiological signs?
- What blood tests would be most useful?

ANSWER 1

The diagnosis is acute haematogenous osteomyelitis. Septic arthritis is less likely in view of the excellent range of movement. There are two principal types of acute osteomyelitis:

- haematogenous osteomyelitis
- direct or contiguous inoculation osteomyelitis.

Acute haematogenous osteomyelitis is characterized by an acute infection of the bone caused by the seeding of the bacteria within the bone from a remote source. This condition occurs primarily in children. The most common site is the rapidly growing and highly vascular metaphysis of growing bones. Direct or contiguous inoculation osteomyelitis is caused by direct contact of the tissue and bacteria during trauma or surgery. Clinical manifestations are more localized and tend to involve multiple organisms.

Predisposing comorbidities include diabetes mellitus, sickle cell disease, acquired immune deficiency syndrome (AIDS), intravenous drug abuse, alcoholism, chronic steroid use, immunosuppression, and chronic joint disease. Other possibilities are the presence of a prosthetic orthopaedic device, recent orthopaedic surgery or an open fracture.

In general, osteomyelitis has a bimodal age distribution. Acute haematogenous osteomyelitis is primarily a disease in children. Direct trauma and contiguous focus osteomyelitis are more common among adults and adolescents than in children. Spinal osteomyelitis is more common in individuals older than 45 years.

The bacterial pathogen varies on the basis of the patient's age and the mechanism of infection:

- in neonates (<4 months) – *Staphylococcus aureus*, *Enterobacter* spp, and group A and B *Streptococcus* spp
- in children (4 months to 4 years) – *S. aureus*, group A *Streptococcus* spp, *Haemophilus influenzae* and *Enterobacter* spp
- in children and adolescents (4 years to adult) – *S. aureus* (80 per cent), group A *Streptococcus* spp, *H. influenzae* and *Enterobacter* spp
- in adults – *S. aureus* and occasionally *Enterobacter* or *Streptococcus* spp.

Responsible pathogens may be isolated in only 35–40 per cent of infections.

With direct osteomyelitis the organisms include *S. aureus*, *Enterobacter* spp and *Pseudomonas* spp. In the presence of puncture wounds there may be *S. aureus* and *Pseudomonas* spp; and in the presence of sickle cell disease, *S. aureus* and *Salmonella* spp.

Appropriate antibiotics are selected using direct culture results. Empirical therapy is often initiated on the basis of the patient's age and the clinical presentation. Further surgical management may involve removal of the nidus of infection and implantation of antibiotic beads until resolution of the infection.

Plain radiographs may show evidence of soft-tissue swelling after 3–5 days. Bony changes are usually present at 14–21 days. The earliest bony changes are periosteal elevation followed by cortical or medullary lucencies. At 28 days, 90 per cent of patients demonstrate some abnormality. Magnetic resonance imaging (MRI) is effective in the early detection of osteomyelitis with a sensitivity ranging from 90 to 100 per cent. Radionuclide bone scanning using a 3-phase bone scan with technetium-99m may show up increased tracer uptake in the affected region. Additional information can be obtained from scanning with leucocytes labelled with gallium-67 and/or indium-111. Computed tomography (CT) scanning can demonstrate calcification, ossification, and intracortical abnormalities. CT is particularly helpful in the evaluation of spinal vertebral lesions. Ultrasonography is useful in children with acute osteomyelitis. This modality can detect abnormalities as early as 1–2 days after onset of symptoms. The abnormalities include soft-tissue abscess or fluid collection and periosteal elevation.

The white cell count may be elevated, but it is frequently normal. The C-reactive protein level is usually elevated, but this is non-specific. The erythrocyte sedimentation rate (ESR) is elevated in 90 per cent, but this finding is clinically non-specific. Blood culture results are positive in only 50 per cent of patients with haematogenous osteomyelitis. Culture or aspiration findings in samples of the infected site are normal in 25 per cent of cases.

 KEY POINTS

- Osteomyelitis can be a result of haematogenous or direct spread.
- The earliest radiographic change is periosteal elevation.
- MRI is effective in the early detection of osteomyelitis.
- The bacterial pathogen varies on the basis of the patient's age and mechanism of infection.

CASE 2: ATRAUMATIC PAINFUL JOINTS IN A BOY

History

A 10-year-old boy has been brought to the emergency department by his father. The youngster was in a playground when he developed a swollen and painful right knee. The boy describes recurrent episodes of pain and swelling in his knees and shoulders over the last year or so. He cannot remember any history of trauma. He does, however, have a history of multiple blood transfusions but he is unsure of the reason for these.

Examination

The boy has painful, tensely swollen, warm and diffusely tender knee and shoulder joints (Fig. 2.1). He also has multiple bruises over his legs and arms.

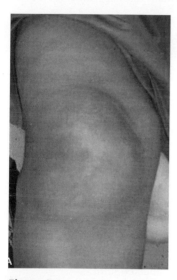

Figure 2.1

Questions

- What is the diagnosis?
- What are the causes of this condition?
- What is the pathophysiology of joint involvement in this condition?

ANSWER 2

This youngster suffers from recurrent episodes of atraumatic painful effusions to his knee joints. He also has a history of multiple blood transfusions. He suffers from a blood dyscrasia leading to haemarthrosis. The most common condition seen in orthopaedic practice is haemophilia and it is most likely in this patient.

Haemophilic arthropathy is a condition associated with a clotting disorder leading to recurrent bleeding into the joints. Over time this can lead to joint destruction. Individuals with haemophilias A and B most commonly have haemophilic arthropathy. Haemophilia A (classic haemophilia) is associated with a factor VIII deficiency and is a sex-linked recessive trait. This occurs in approximately 1 per 5000 live male births, with 25 per cent of cases being sporadic (no family history). Other clotting disorders may also lead to haemarthrosis, examples being haemophilia B (Christmas disease) and factor IX deficiency.

Haemosiderin deposition within the joint leads to synovial hypertrophy, bone erosions, recurrent bleeding, and eventual destruction of the articular surfaces and arthrofibrosis. The stages of degenerative changes in the joint are summarized below.

! **Stages of joint changes with haemarthrosis**

- Grade 1: Soft-tissue swelling (effusions, synovial thickening)
- Grade 2: Widened epiphysis, small erosions (normal cartilage interval)
- Grade 3: Large erosions, bone cysts, cartilage loss
- Grade 4: Joint destruction and subluxation

KEY POINTS

- Haemosiderin deposition within the joint leads to synovial hypertrophy, bone erosions and recurrent bleeding.
- Recurrent haemarthrosis can lead to joint destruction of the affected joints.
- Synovectomy should be considered, or replace or fuse the joint.

CASE 3: AN ATRAUMATIC PAINFUL HIP

History

A 32-year-old Afro-Caribbean man was intending to visit his mother in Africa. While packing he noticed a progressively worsening pain in the left groin. The pain radiated down the upper thigh and was present at rest. There were no aggravating or relieving factors and no associated symptoms of numbness or tingling. The pain was severe and constant in nature for several days. He had also noticed some mild discomfort in his left hip. He recalls no previous episodes. He obtained temporary relief of his pain with simple analgesia. He has a history of asthma and has been taking regular steroids over the last 15 years. He drinks 20 units of alcohol per week and smokes 20 cigarettes a day. There is no history of trauma and he is systemically well.

Examination

The man walks with a severe limp. Assessment of his hip abductors reveals a positive Trendelenburg sign on the left side. Measurement of the true leg lengths reveals a 1 cm shortening in the left leg compared to the right. Movement of the hip is painful but not significantly restricted. He has no obvious neurological or vascular deficit of the legs. A radiograph of this patient is shown in Fig. 3.1.

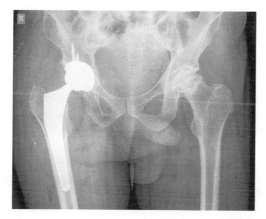

Figure 3.1

Questions

- What is the diagnosis?
- Describe the blood supply to the femoral head.
- What factors predispose to this condition?
- How would you investigate and classify this condition?
- What are the management options?

ANSWER 3

This man has insidious and persistent left groin pain that is exacerbated by weight-bearing. This pain arises from his hip joint. While he retains a good range of movement, he has pain. He also has true leg shortening. He has mild symptoms in the right hip. Finally, he has a history of being on steroids and is a heavy smoker and consumes alcohol. All these signs indicate that the most likely diagnosis is avascular necrosis of the femoral head. This is the most common site to undergo avascular necrosis. The condition is bilateral in 50 per cent of patients. Around 10 per cent are asymptomatic and diagnosed incidentally.

The blood supply to the femoral head is derived from an arterial ring around the neck of femur. The ring anastomosis is mainly from the medial femoral circumflex artery posteriorly and minor branches of the lateral femoral circumflex artery anteriorly. These vessels traverse the femoral neck to perforate the head close to the articular cartilage. Ten per cent of the blood supply comes from the vessels in the ligamentum teres.

An injury or ischaemia can predispose to arterial cut-off, venous stasis, intravascular thrombosis, intraosseus sinusoidal compression or a combination of these. The decreased blood flow to the femoral head leads to increased intraosseus pressure, osteonecrosis and finally collapse of the femoral head.

Traumatic causes of avascular necrosis of the femoral head are fracture of neck of femur and dislocation of the femoral head. Non-traumatic causes include steroid use, alcoholism, marrow-replacing diseases like Gaucher's disease, high-dose radiotherapy, hypercoagulable states, sickle cell disease, hyperfibrinolysis, thrombophilia, protein C and S deficiency, and Legg–Calvé–Perthes disease (LCPD).

Imaging the hip with anteroposterior and lateral views is the initial investigation. In early cases the radiographs may not reveal any signs of avascular necrosis. In late cases, subchondral sclerosis (increased density of the affected area, crescent sign), a thin subchondral fracture line in the necrotic segment, flattening of the femoral head, and collapse of the femoral head can be seen. The important differentiating point from advanced osteoarthritis is the preservation of joint space during the early stages of the disease.

MRI scans are the investigation of choice in patients with normal radiographs. They can show early changes in the bone marrow long before the appearance of X-ray features.

There are a number of classifications for avascular necrosis of the femoral head. The most commonly used classification was described by Ficat and associates in 1960, based on radiological findings and bone scans.

! **The Ficat classification**

Pre-collapse phase
- Ficat I: No X-ray changes
- Ficat II: Early X-ray changes, no distortion of femoral head

Post-collapse phase
- Ficat III: Increased bone destruction, femoral head deformed on X-ray
- Ficat IV: Complete collapse of femoral head with destruction of hip joint seen on X-ray

---

Management depends on the stage of disease seen at first presentation. If early avascular necrosis is left untreated it is likely to progress to the advanced stages. Management of pre-collapse avascular necrosis comprises surgical intervention with core decompression with or without bone grafts.

KEY POINTS

- The femoral head is the most common site to undergo avascular necrosis.
- The condition is bilateral in 50 per cent of cases.
- Traumatic and atraumatic causes have been identified.
- Radiographs may be normal in the early stages.
- MRI is the investigation of choice.
- Treatment options include core decompression and bone graft, osteotomy and arthroplasty.

CASE 4: AN EXPANDING MASS IN THE LEG OF AN ADOLESCENT

History

A 15-year-old boy was on holiday abroad with his parents. While sunbathing the boy asked his father to apply suntan lotion to his legs. The father then noticed a lump over the proximal aspect of his son's tibia that was not present on the other leg. The boy explained that the lump had been there for nearly 6 months but had been increasing in size over the recent few weeks. The family immediately returned home to consult their doctor.

Examination

On inspection there is a firm, irregular and tender mass arising from the proximal tibia. The boy describes no pain on palpation of the lump and his range of movement is full. There are no other lumps. Radiographs of his knee are shown in Figs 4.1 and 4.2. His erythrocyte sedimentation rate (ESR) and serum alkaline phosphatase are raised.

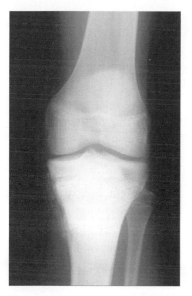 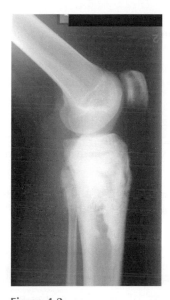

Figure 4.1   Figure 4.2

Questions

- What is the diagnosis?
- Describe the features of the X-rays.
- How would you confirm the diagnosis?
- What are the principles of management of this condition?

ANSWER 4

This boy has an osteosarcoma of the proximal tibia. A firm, irregular mass fixed to underlying structures is more suspicious of a malignant lesion. This is a malignant tumour of the proximal tibia. This is the most common primary malignant bone tumour of mesenchymal derivation. The tumour arises in adolescents and affects males more often than females. The most common site affected is in the region of the knee in the metaphyseal part of the bone. Other sites include the proximal humerus, proximal femur and pelvis, and the spine is rarely involved.

Osteosarcoma can present as purely osteolytic or osteoblastic or a mixture of the two types. Elevation of the periosteum may appear as a classic Codman's triangle. Near the junction of the healthy bone with the tumour there is reactive new bone formation beneath the periosteum as seen in the proximal tibia in this case. Extension of the tumour through the periosteum may produce a sunburst appearance which is also present in the X-rays. Remember always to image the entire bone to assess for skip lesions or joint involvement.

A biopsy of the lesion will help confirm the diagnosis. The biopsy should be undertaken ideally by the same surgeon who will be responsible for the definitive tumour resection in a dedicated bone and soft-tissue sarcoma unit. Biopsies performed without communication with the dedicated sarcoma unit's input can lead to amputation of a salvageable limb.

The Enneking staging system is the most widely used. The key components in staging are histological grade (low-grade vs high-grade), the anatomical location of the tumour (intracompartmental vs extracompartmental), and the presence or absence of metastatic disease.

Management comprises staging of the tumour, neo-adjuvant treatment, and surgery in a specialist bone and soft-tissue sarcoma unit with a multidisciplinary team.

Most patients have micrometastases at the time of presentation. All should be screened for pulmonary metastasis. The principle of treatment is, therefore, to combine surgery (limb salvage or amputation) with chemotherapy. Limb salvage is possible only if the nerves can be preserved, adequate muscles and soft tissues can be left intact while a reasonably wide margin of resection of the tumour can be achieved. Radiotherapy is usually reserved for palliation and disease location in an inaccessible location. Pre- and postoperative chemotherapy is used for osteosarcoma. Patients with a greater than 95 per cent tumour cell kill or necrosis have a better prognosis than those whose tumours do not respond as favourably. With adjuvant chemotherapy, the 5-year survival rate can be greater than 50 per cent.

KEY POINTS
• Osteosarcoma is the most common primary malignant bone tumour of mesenchymal derivation.   • The most common site affected is in the region of the knee.   • MRI of the primary lesion is the best method to use.   • Biopsy of the lesion will help confirm the diagnosis.   • Management comprises staging of the tumour, neo-adjuvant treatment, and surgery in a specialist unit.

CASE 5: A BOY WITH A SWOLLEN MASS IN HIS THIGH

History

A 14-year-old boy presents to his general practitioner with a swelling around the mid shaft of his femur. His mother has brought him in following his complaints of tiredness and intermittent fevers over the last few weeks, which has caused him to miss football training and to be inactive.

Examination

Manual examination of the mid thigh reveals a tender mass. The mass is firm and appears to be well fixed to the underlying muscle. There are no neurological or vascular deficits to the leg. Initial investigations reveal elevated white blood cells (WBC), erythrocyte sedimentation rate (ESR) and anaemia. A radiograph of the femur is shown in Fig. 5.1.

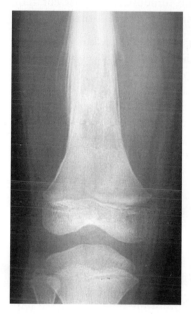

Figure 5.1

Questions

- What is the diagnosis?
- Describe the features of the X-ray.
- How would you manage this condition?
- What is the prognosis?

ANSWER 5

The diagnosis is Ewing's sarcoma. The features suspicious of a malignant lesion in this age group are the firm, fixed mass, its location, and raised inflammatory markers associated with anaemia, fatigue and intermittent fevers. This condition typically occurs in young patients and presents with pain and fever.

The tumour was first described by James Ewing in 1921 and is the second most common primary malignant bone tumour (the first being osteosarcoma). The tumour is more common in males and affects children and young adults. The majority develop this between the ages of 10 and 20 years. Rarely, the tumour develops in adults older than 30 years.

The earliest symptom is pain, which is initially intermittent but becomes intense. Rarely, a patient may present with a pathological fracture. Eighty-five per cent of patients have chromosomal translocations associated with the 11/22 chromosome. Ewing's sarcoma is potentially the most aggressive form of the primary bone tumours. The most common sites affected are the femoral diaphysis, pelvis, tibia, humerus, fibula and ribs.

Radiological features seen in the femoral shaft include a typical onion-skin appearance or sunburst pattern due to spread of the tumour via Haversian canals with periosteal reaction which indicates an aggressive process. In some patients, Codman triangles may be present at the margins of the lesion. These result from the elevation of the periosteum and central destruction of the periosteal reaction caused by the tumour. Radiographs may vary from highly lytic to predominantly sclerotic in appearance. Most commonly, radiographs show a long, permeative lytic lesion in the meta-diaphysis and diaphysis of the bone. Sclerotic lesions are less common. MRI provides a more accurate assessment of the tumour size and relation to the surrounding structures.

Patients are usually assigned to one of two groups, the tumour being classified as either localized or metastatic disease. Tumours in the pelvis typically present late and are therefore larger with a poorer prognosis. Treatment comprises chemotherapy, surgical resection and/or radiotherapy. With combined treatment, patient survival has improved: with the use of adjuvant chemotherapy, the 5-year survival rate is more than 60 per cent. With localized disease, wide surgical excision of the tumour is preferred over radiotherapy if the involved bone is expendable (e.g. fibular, rib), or if radiotherapy would damage the growth plate. If there is a pathological fracture, limb salvage surgery with the implantation of a long mega-prosthesis is the preferred option.

Non-metastatic disease survival rates are 55–70 per cent, compared to 22–33 per cent for metastatic disease. Patients require careful follow-up owing to the risk of developing osteosarcoma following radiotherapy, particularly in children in whom it can occur in up to 20 per cent of cases. A European study of 359 patients with non-metastatic Ewing's sarcoma revealed that the following factors are associated with a poor prognosis:

- male sex
- age >12 years
- anaemia
- elevated lactate dehydrogenase (LDH)
- radiation therapy only for local control
- poor chemotherapeutic course.

KEY POINTS

- The majority of cases of Ewing's tumour are seen between the ages of 10 and 20 years.
- Eighty-five per cent of patients have chromosomal translocations associated with chromosome 11/22.
- Most common sites affected are the femoral diaphysis, pelvis, tibia, humerus, fibula and ribs.
- Radiological features include an onion-skin appearance or sunburst.
- Treatment comprises chemotherapy, surgical resection and/or radiotherapy.

CASE 6: A PAINFUL COLLARBONE

History

A 25-year-old triathlete fell from his cycle while training and landed on his left shoulder. He was wearing a helmet. When he tried to pick up his cycle he felt severe pain in his left collarbone and was unable to pick up the machine. He has presented to the emergency department.

Examination

The man has some swelling and deformity in the region of the middle of the collarbone. On palpation he feels pain and tenderness over the left collarbone. The upper ribs are not tender. The overlying skin is intact, and there is no evidence of any neurological or vascular deficit of either arm. A radiograph is shown in Fig. 6.1.

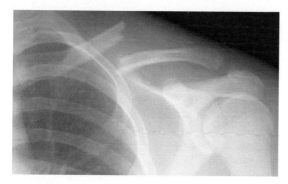

Figure 6.1

Questions
- What is the diagnosis?
- Can you classify these injuries?
- What imaging views do you need to describe these injuries?
- How would you manage this patient?

ANSWER 6

The diagnosis is a fractured clavicle. This is a common fracture following direct trauma. Anatomically, the acromioclavicular and coracoclavicular ligaments attach the clavicle to the scapula laterally. The sternoclavicular and the costoclavicular ligaments anchor the clavicle medially. The sternocleidomastoid and the subclavius muscles also have points of attachment to the clavicle. The clavicle also protects the adjacent brachial plexus, lung and blood vessels.

The most popular classification divides the clavicle into thirds: medial, middle and lateral. This case is a middle-third fracture.

Medial-third injuries are rare and account for only 5 per cent of clavicle fractures because very strong forces are required to cause fracture in this area. They may be associated with intrathoracic injuries or the development of late complications, such as arthritis.

Middle-third fractures occur medial to the coracoclavicular ligament, at the junction of the middle and outer thirds of the clavicle. The usual mechanism of injury involves a direct force applied to the lateral aspect of the shoulder. Most middle-third fractures in both adults and children will heal without surgical intervention. The medial fragment displaces upwards due to the pull of the sternocleidomastoid muscle. The lateral fragment displaces downwards due to the weight of the limb.

Lateral-third fractures account for 10–15 per cent of clavicle fractures and may go on to non-union. These fractures result from a direct blow to the top of the shoulder. They occur distal to the coracoclavicular ligament and are classified further into three subtypes. Type 1 fractures are undisplaced, and the coracoclavicular ligaments remain intact. Type 2 fractures are displaced, and there is associated rupture of the coracoclavicular ligament with the proximal clavicular segment typically pulled upward by the sternocleidomastoid muscle. Type 3 injuries involve the articular surface of the acromioclavicular joint.

Appropriate imaging views are anteroposterior and beam-angled 30 degrees cephalad. A thorough assessment to exclude the presence of a scapular fracture should be made. In the presence of a scapular fracture as well as a clavicle fracture, this would represent a floating shoulder.

Most undisplaced mid-shaft fractures are treated non-operatively. Union usually occurs and produces prominent callus. A broad arm sling for 2–6 weeks is commonly recommended. Patients should be advised to discard the sling once the acute pain settles, encouraging shoulder range of motion and normal activities as comfort allows. However, distal clavicle fractures have a higher incidence of non-union. The majority of these are asymptomatic and a few will be severe enough to require fixation. Shortening of 1.5–2 cm may lead to residual symptoms related to the shoulder and unsatisfactory outcome.

Operative treatment should be considered in adults with significantly displaced, high-energy, multi-fragmentary, shortened mid-shaft fractures (>1.5–2 cm), vertical fragment, open fracture, or when the skin is imminently threatened, associated floating shoulder and neurovascular compromise. With surgery, consider fixation with a contoured plate and screws. Plate removal following union may be necessary if the plate is prominent. Contact sport should be avoided until the bone healing is solid.

KEY POINTS

- Clavicle fractures occur following direct trauma.
- Most undisplaced mid-shaft fractures are treated non-operatively.
- Lateral-third fractures have a higher rate of non-union.
- Surgery comprises plate fixation.

CASE 7: A PAINFUL PROXIMAL HUMERUS IN AN ELDERLY WOMAN

History

An 85-year-old woman suffered a fall while shopping in icy conditions in winter. She landed on her shoulder. Immediately she complained of severe pain and suspected her shoulder was starting to swell. She has been taken to the local emergency department, where she continues to complain of severe pain in her right shoulder. She has a past medical history of hypertension treated with bendroflumethiazide, but has been otherwise well.

Examination

There is a large bruise and swelling over the right shoulder, extending down to the proximal one-third of the humerus, as well as tenderness to palpation over the right shoulder girdle. She can hardly move her right arm because of the pain. There is no neurovascular deficit. Radiographs are shown in Figs 7.1and 7.2.

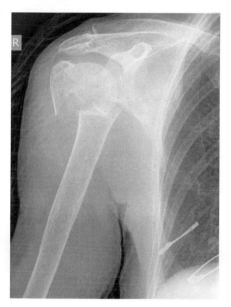

Figure 7.1

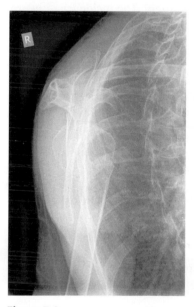

Figure 7.2

Questions

- What is the diagnosis?
- Describe the relevant anatomy.
- How would you manage this patient?

ANSWER 7

This is a fracture of the proximal humerus. The X-rays show displacement of the greater tuberosity and the surgical neck of humerus. The humeral head is not dislocated. This is a typical fracture pattern in an elderly woman with osteoporosis. Swelling and tenderness to palpation are typically present. Bruising extending along the arm distally and along the chest wall is often present a few days following injury.

The proximal humerus consists of four bony parts: humeral head (articular surface), greater tuberosity, lesser tuberosity and the humeral diaphysis. Radiographs should include anteroposterior, lateral and axillary views, and often a CT reconstruction scan to assess the fragments involved.

Fracture stability can be assessed by placing one hand on the humeral head while gently rotating the humeral shaft internally and externally. If the proximal and distal fragments move as a unit, the fracture is considered stable.

A neurovascular examination is essential owing to the proximity of the brachial plexus and axillary artery. The incidence of neurovascular injury is increased in fracture dislocations. The axillary nerve is most commonly injured.

Indications for open or closed reduction and internal fixation are related to the fracture pattern, the quality of the bone, the status of the rotator cuff, and the age and activity level of the patient. The goal of reduction and fixation of a proximal humeral fracture is to obtain nearly anatomical reduction and stable fixation to allow an early range of motion. Undisplaced fractures are treated conservatively.

Most of the displaced one- or two-part fractures are treated with closed reduction and pin fixation or open reduction and internal fixation. The treatment options for three-part proximal humerus fractures include proximal humeral plate and screws or proximal humeral intramedullary nail. The preferred treatment of four-part fractures is humeral head replacement if fixation with a plate and screws is not possible. This is primarily because of the high risk of osteonecrosis and secondarily because of the difficulty in obtaining secure internal fixation.

 KEY POINTS

- The incidence of neurovascular injury is increased in fracture dislocations of the proximal humerus.
- The axillary nerve is most commonly injured.
- Blood supply to the humerus is predominantly via the anterior humeral circumflex artery.
- Muscle attachments when a fracture occurs produce deforming forces.
- Treatment options include conservative, open reduction and internal fixation and hemiarthroplasty.

CASE 8: A BOY WITH A PAINFUL ELBOW

History

A 7-year-old boy fell from his bicycle and described landing on his outstretched right arm in abduction with the elbow in extension. He complained immediately of severe pain around the right elbow, but no other parts of his body were painful. He has presented to the emergency department.

Examination

Inspection of his right elbow reveals some swelling. On palpation of the elbow, he has most tenderness across the lateral aspect of his distal right humerus. This tenderness is associated with a significant reduced range of motion of the elbow flexion and extension. He has no neurovascular deficit of the arm. A radiograph is shown in Fig. 8.1.

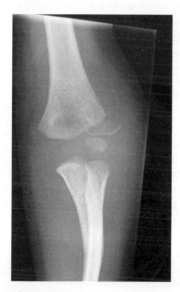

Figure 8.1

Questions

- What is the diagnosis?
- How would you classify this condition?
- How would you manage this patient?

ANSWER 8

This boy has a fracture of the lateral condyle of the humerus. The fracture line extends from the diaphysis and epiphysis which communicate through the growth plate. The lateral condyle fracture is a Salter–Harris type IV pattern. These fractures most commonly occur at ages between 6 and 10 years.

Fractures of the lateral condyle of the humerus are unstable. The distal humerus is predominantly cartilage at this age and knowledge of the secondary centres of ossification is helpful to understand the fracture patterns. Fractures therefore often appear subtle on the radiographs because most of the fracture line courses through the cartilage and is not seen on plain radiographs.

Milch in 1956 classified these lateral humeral condyle fractures as types I and II. These subgroups are based on the location of the fracture line. A Milch type I fracture exits through the ossification centre of the lateral condyle and exits at the radiocapitellar groove. This pattern is least common. A Milch type II fracture extends into the apex of the trochlea, which produces elbow instability, and is the more common fracture pattern. In this case, the fracture has a tendency to dislocate laterally and so should be treated surgically.

Lateral condyle fractures with less than 2 mm of displacement may be treated with immobilization in an above-elbow plaster for approximately 3 weeks followed by gentle mobilization. Close follow-up is necessary to look out for fracture displacement. Operative management is essential for all displaced fractures, as in the present case. An arthrogram assesses the size of the cartilaginous fragment and the degree of articular displacement which can help in decision-making in difficult cases. Fragment stabilization is most frequently performed using two percutaneously placed smooth Kirschner wires (k-wires). If the fracture is grossly unstable, open reduction and stabilization with wires may be necessary. Care must be taken during the exposure to avoid denuding the blood supply to the lateral condyle from the posterior soft-tissue structure. Following fixation, an above-elbow plaster is applied with the forearm in supination. At 3–4 weeks, the k-wires are removed and follow-up scheduled at 6 weeks for further X-rays. A return to full activity is allowed once the fracture has united radiographically.

 KEY POINTS

- Humeral condyle fractures occur most commonly between 6 and 10 years of age. The distal humerus is predominantly cartilage at this stage of development.
- Fractures often appear subtle on radiographs.
- Displacement of less than 2 mm can be treated with immobilization in a cast. Operative management is essential for all other displaced fractures.
- Monitor growth radiographically up to skeletal maturity.

CASE 9: A PAINFUL DISTAL RADIUS FOLLOWING A FALL

History

An 85-year-old woman was walking her dog in the early morning. She slipped on ice and fell, landing directly on her outstretched hand. She immediately felt a crack in her wrist and then pain. She noticed some swelling appear around the distal radius and experienced some pins and needles in her thumb, index finger and middle finger. She called for help and has been taken to the emergency department for assessment.

Examination

This elderly woman's wrist reveals marked swelling. The distal radius appears to have a dinner-fork type deformity. On palpation of the wrist, she has severe tenderness of the distal radius. She is very reluctant to move her wrist in any direction because of the pain. Assessment of her sensation reveals altered sensation in her thumb and index and middle fingers, but she is still able to move her thumb. The radius and ulna pulses are palpable. A radiograph is shown in Fig. 9.1.

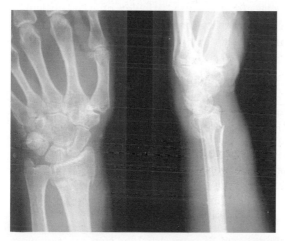

Figure 9.1

Questions
- What is the diagnosis?
- What are the risk factors for this injury?
- How would you classify these injuries?
- How would you manage this patient?

ANSWER 9

The X-ray shows an extra-articular fracture of the distal radius. There is some dorsal angulation of the distal fragment and radial shortening. The diagnosis is thus a distal radius fracture.

These injuries were first described by an Irish surgeon, Abraham Colles, in 1814, and are commonly called Colles' fractures. His description was based on clinical examination alone because X-rays had not been invented. Distal radius fractures are the most common fractures. Colles' fractures account for over 90 per cent of distal radius fractures. Any injury to the median nerve can produce paraesthesia in the thumb, index finger, and middle and radial border of the ring finger – as in this case.

There is a bimodal age distribution of fractures to the distal radius with two peaks occurring. The first peak occurs in people aged 18–25 years, and a second peak in older people (>65 years). High-energy injuries are more common in the younger group and low-energy injuries in the older group. Osteoporosis may play a role in the occurrence of this later fracture. In the group of patients between 60 and 69 years, women far outnumber men.

Broadly, distal radius fractures can be classified as intra-articular or extra-articular. Eponyms have been added to the various sub-classifications, examples being Smith fractures, Barton fractures and volar Barton fractures.

Management aims to restore the patient's functioning to the pre-injury level. This can be achieved by restoration of the radial shortening, radial inclination and dorsal angulation. Assessment with plain radiographs is all that is needed for most fractures. CT scans, however, are useful for evaluating the articular fracture lines and degree of comminution, and they are sometimes useful for planning the surgical approach.

The majority of distal radius fractures can be treated conservatively. With fractures that are minimally displaced, a forearm cast is worn for 6 weeks. Note that elderly, low-activity patients can have satisfactory function even with a significantly displaced fracture, although they may have a residual dinner-fork wrist deformity (due to a prominent ulna head) that has limited supination and flexion.

Most surgeons would not accept more than 2 mm of intra-articular step-off, not more than 10 degrees of dorsal tilt (although some surgeons only accept no more than neutral) and 2 mm of radial shortening. Shortening of more than 2 mm doubles the load through the triangular fibrocartilage and the ulna. The surgical options include fixation with percutaneous wires, open reduction and internal fixation, or external fixators.

 KEY POINTS

- Colles' fractures account for over 90 per cent of distal radius fractures.
- There is a bimodal age distribution of fractures.
- Distal radius fractures can be classified as intra-articular or extra-articular types.
- Treatment for a minimally displaced fracture is a forearm cast. Surgical options for displaced fractures are fixation with wire or plate and screws.

CASE 10: A PAINFUL THUMB FOLLOWING A FALL

History

A 22-year-old man was on a skiing holiday when he accidentally landed on the ground with his hand braced on a ski pole. He complained of immediate pain and swelling at the base of his thumb following a valgus force being placed onto his abducted metacarpo-phalangeal joint. He has attended the local hospital for assessment.

Examination

He has some swelling at the base of his thumb. On palpation he complains of tenderness over his thumb carpometacarpal joint, particularly over the ulnar border. He demonstrates reduced range of movement in his thumb. A radiograph is shown in Fig. 10.1.

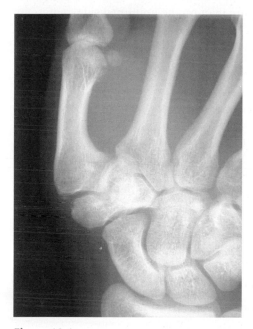

Figure 10.1

Questions

- What is the diagnosis?
- What investigation is useful in addition to the X-ray?
- What is a Stener lesion?
- How would you manage this injury?

ANSWER 10

The diagnosis is 'gamekeeper's thumb' because the valgus force placed onto the abducted metacarpophalangeal (MCP) joint leads to an ulnar collateral ligament injury (UCL). Campbell originally coined the term 'gamekeeper's thumb' in 1955, because this condition was most commonly associated with Scottish gamekeepers. This injury results in instability, pain and weakness of the pinch grasp. To assess for instability the thumb should be examined by placing it in 30-degree flexion and tested for valgus instability.

The UCL originates from the metacarpal head and inserts into the medial aspect and base of the proximal phalanx of the thumb. Occasionally, when the UCL is strained, it avulses the bone at its insertion and leads to a gamekeeper's fracture. Although a gamekeeper's fracture is a contraindication to stress testing, an undisplaced avulsion fracture is not. If the patient's pain is severe, the joint may be anaesthetized locally with an injection. A laxity of 30 degrees, or one that is 15 degrees more than on the uninjured side, represents a ruptured collateral ligament in this position. If valgus laxity of the MCP joint is present in both the flexed and extended positions, complete UCL rupture should be suspected.

Ultrasound is 92 per cent sensitive for UCL ruptures and provides a positive predictive value of 99 per cent.

A Stener lesion occurs when the adductor aponeurosis becomes interposed between the ruptured UCL and its site of insertion at the base of the proximal phalanx. The distal portion of the ligament retracts and points superficially and proximally. A rupture of the proper and accessory collateral ligaments must occur for this injury to happen. The UCL therefore no longer contacts its area of insertion and cannot heal. Occasionally, the UCL avulses a small portion of the proximal phalanx at its insertion, leading to a gamekeeper's fracture.

Non-surgical treatment can be considered for partial tears of the UCL; that is, grade I or grade II tears as in this case. The thumb is immobilized in a spica-type cast for 4 weeks. The cast should be well-moulded around the MCP joint, and the interphalangeal (IP) joint can be left free. If the fragment is displaced by less than 2 mm, non-surgical management is indicated. For greater displacement, the fracture should be opened and reduced. Complete ulnar collateral ligament tears require surgical repair.

 KEY POINTS

- A valgus force placed on an MCP joint leads to an ulnar collateral ligament injury.
- A Stener lesion occurs when the adductor aponeurosis becomes interposed between the ruptured UCL and its site of insertion at the base of the proximal phalanx.
- Ultrasound is 92 per cent sensitive for UCL ruptures.
- Non-surgical treatment can be considered for partial tears. For greater displacement, the fracture should be opened and reduced.

CASE 11: A PAINFUL HIP FOLLOWING A FALL

History

A 72-year-old woman tripped, fell and landed on her left hip. She reported pain in her proximal thigh and was unable to bear weight. An ambulance was called and she has been taken to the emergency department.

Examination

This elderly woman is in some obvious pain which appears to be arising from her hip. She has evidence of shortening of the left leg and the leg is lying in external rotation. There is significant swelling and tenderness to palpation in the proximal thigh region. This is a closed injury and she has no neurovascular deficit. A radiograph is shown in Fig. 11.1.

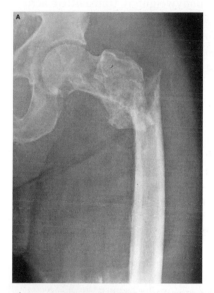

Figure 11.1

Questions

- What is the diagnosis?
- What is a potential secondary cause of this injury?
- Describe the anatomy of the proximal femur and the effect the muscles have on this injury.
- How would you manage this type of injury?

ANSWER 11

The diagnosis is a subtrochanteric fracture, because the fracture seen on the anteroposterior X-ray is below the level of the lesser trochanter. Subtrochanteric fractures account for about 10–30 per cent of all hip fractures. These fractures typically are seen in two patient groups: older osteopenic patients after a low-energy fall, and younger patients involved in high-energy trauma.

In the older group, falls are the most frequent mechanism of injury. Importantly, this age group is particularly susceptible to metastatic disease that can lead to pathological fractures.

The subtrochanteric region of the femur, arbitrarily designated as the region between the lesser trochanter and a point 5 cm distal, consists predominantly of cortical bone. During normal activities of daily living, up to six times the bodyweight is transmitted across the subtrochanteric region of the femur. The lesser trochanter is posteromedial, and it is the point of insertion for the psoas and iliacus tendons. The femoral shaft has both an anterior and a lateral bow. The major muscles that surround the hip create significant forces that contribute to fracture deformity. The gluteus medius and gluteus minimus tendons attach to the greater trochanter and abduct the proximal fragment. The psoas and iliacus attach to the lesser trochanter and flex the proximal fragment – as in this case. The adductors pull the distal fragment medially.

Intramedullary nails are emerging as the treatment of choice for subtrochanteric femur fractures. For some fractures with extension above the lesser trochanter, a fixed-angle device such as a blade-plate or dynamic condylar screw can be considered as surgical options. In the presence of pathological fractures, prophylactic stabilization of the entire femur may be indicated to prevent problems with multiple metastases in the same bone.

 KEY POINTS

- There are two patient groups, namely older osteopenic patients after a low-energy fall and younger patients involved in high-energy trauma.
- The subtrochanteric region is between the lesser trochanter and a point 5 cm distal.
- Intramedullary nails are emerging as the treatment of choice.

CASE 12: KNEE PAIN FOLLOWING A TRAFFIC ACCIDENT

History

A 70-year-old man was driving his car along a main road when another vehicle pulled out of a side street and collided with his vehicle. After the impact he complained of pain in the superior aspect of his right knee. An ambulance came to the scene and took him to the emergency department.

Examination

This elderly man has a closed injury and swelling in the distal aspect of the femur and knee. He has some obvious tenderness to palpation around the distal femur. Radiographs of his injury are shown in Figs 12.1 and 12.2.

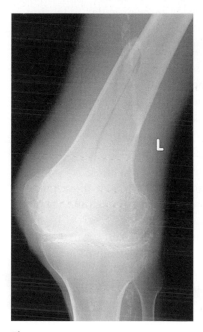

Figure 12.1

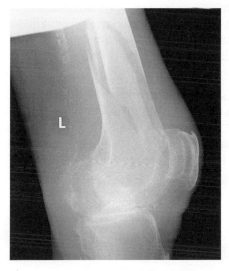

Figure 12.2

Questions

- What is the diagnosis?
- Which radiographs would you request for this injury?
- What are the principles of management of this kind of injury?

ANSWER 12

The diagnosis is a supracondylar femoral fracture. The anteroposterior and lateral X-rays show multiple fracture lines within the distal femur consistent with a shortened and displaced fracture. These injuries make up 6 per cent of all femoral fractures. There is a bimodal distribution of fractures based on age and gender. Most high-energy distal femur fractures occur in males aged between 15 and 50 years, while most low-energy fractures occur in osteoporotic women aged 50 or above. The most common high-energy mechanism of injury is a road traffic accident (RTA), and the most common low-energy mechanism is a fall.

Depending on the mechanism of injury, radiographic evaluation of distal femur fractures may include orthogonal plain radiographs of the entire length of the femur to avoid missing ipsilateral femoral neck or shaft fractures. True knee radiographs are required to screen for intra-articular extension of fracture lines. If intra-articular extension is suspected – particularly coronal plane fractures which can be difficult to see on plain X-rays – a CT scan may be helpful in planning treatment.

In general, however, non-operative treatment does not work well for displaced fractures. With this patient, operative treatment is indicated. Operative intervention is also indicated in the presence of open fractures and injuries associated with vascular injury. The aim of surgery is to achieve anatomical reduction of the joint surface with stable fixation, restoration of limb alignment, and early postoperative movement of the knee joint. This patient should have an open reduction and internal fixation with a plate and screws.

Multiple options exist for the definitive treatment of distal femur fractures. They include external fixation (for patients with open fractures and bone loss, vascular injury, associated significant soft-tissue injuries, or extensive comminution), intramedullary nailing (for fractures with enough intact distal femur to allow for interlocking screw fixation), and plate osteosynthesis with either open reduction and internal fixation or minimally invasive plate osteosynthesis. Likewise, multiple plating options are available and include conventional buttress plates, fixed-angle devices, and locking plates. Locked implants are typically indicated in patients with osteoporosis, fractures with metaphyseal comminution where the medial cortex cannot be restored, or a short articular segment. Total knee replacement is effective in elderly patients with articular fractures and significant osteoporosis, or pre-existing arthritis that is not amenable to open reduction and internal fixation.

Low-demand elderly patients with non- or minimally displaced fractures can be managed conservatively. The techniques comprise either skeletal traction or initial splinting and mobilization with limited weight-bearing and eventual progression to either a cast or functional brace. Radiographs should be obtained at weekly to bi-weekly intervals for the first 6 weeks to ensure that the fracture reduction is maintained. The patient should gradually progress to weight-bearing, and joint mobilization should be allowed based on the clinical and radiographic progression of fracture healing. In general, this fracture can take a minimum of 3–4 months to unite.

KEY POINTS

- High-energy distal femur fractures occur in males aged between 15 and 50 years. Most low-energy fractures occur in osteoporotic women over the age of 50 years.
- Shortening of the fracture with varus and extension of the distal articular segment is the typical deformity.
- Radiographic evaluation of distal femur fractures may include orthogonal plain radiographs.
- Low-demand elderly patients with non- or minimally displaced fractures can be managed conservatively.
- The aim of surgery in displaced fractures is to achieve anatomical reduction of the joint surface with stable fixation, restoration of limb alignment, and early postoperative movement of the knee joint.

CASE 13: A PAINFUL SWOLLEN ELBOW IN A YOUNG GIRL

History

A 6-year-old girl was playing on a trampoline in a garden when she fell off. She landed on the grass but developed pain and swelling in her elbow immediately. Her mother took her to the emergency department.

Examination

The elbow is markedly swollen and tender in the distal humerus both medially and laterally. The girl is reluctant to move the elbow owing to the pain. Assessment of the neurovascular status of the limb reveals a palpable radial pulse with no neurological compromise. A radiograph is shown in Fig. 13.1.

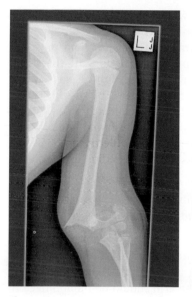

Figure 13.1

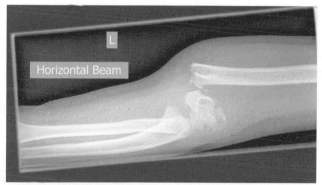

Figure 13.2

Questions

- What is the diagnosis?
- How would you examine this young patient?
- How would you manage her injury?
- What are possible complications of this injury?

ANSWER 13

This young girl has sustained a supracondylar fracture of the humerus. In children this type of fracture remains extra-articular. There are two types of supracondylar fracture: the extension type (95 per cent) and the flexion type (5 per cent). The pattern of the fracture occurs with failure of the anterior cortex first, followed by posterior displacement of the distal fragment. For the extension type injury, Gartland in 1959 classified the injury into three types: type I is undisplaced; type II is displaced with the posterior hinge intact; and type III is completely displaced with no periosteal attachment – as in this case.

A detailed history is necessary to understand the mechanism of injury. A fall onto an outstretched hand may lead to an extension-type fracture, whereas a fall onto the elbow can result in a flexion supracondylar fracture. Prior to the treatment of supracondylar fractures, it is essential to identify the type.

Examination of the degree of swelling and deformity as well as a neurological and vascular status assessment of the forearm is essential. A vascular injury may present with signs of an acute compartment syndrome with pain, paraesthesia, pallor, and pulseless and tight forearm. Injury to the brachial artery may present with loss of the distal pulse. However, in the presence of a weak distal pulse, major vessel injury may still be present owing to the collateral circulation. The most common nerve to sustain injury is the anterior interosseous branch of the median nerve (ask the child to make a circle with the thumb and the index finger: known as the 'okay sign'). The radial, median and ulnar nerves are injured less commonly. The latter may be injured while trying to fix the fracture during insertion of the medial pin. Finally, assess the distal radius for fractures, reported to occur in 5–6 per cent of cases.

Treatment of a type I injury is symptomatic in minimally displaced fractures. Flex the elbow just past 90 degrees and immobilize in a collar and cuff and/or back-slab for 3–4 weeks.

Treatment of a type II injury involves a general anaesthetic. The aim of the manipulation of the fracture is to correct the angulation in the frontal and sagittal planes. The reduction technique comprises elbow pronation and flexion. The arm should be immobilized in pronation and elbow flexion not exceeding 120 degrees. With the elbow flexed beyond 90 degrees the injury should be stable due to an intact posterior periosteal hinge. If the swelling prohibits elbow flexion to 90 degrees, or if excessive flexion is necessary to maintain reduction, then fixation with wires may be necessary to maintain reduction. Gartland type II fractures have been subdivided into two types: IIA and IIB. Type IIA have posterior angulation with an intact posterior cortex/hinge with no rotational deformity; type IIB have some degree of rotational deformity. Type IIB fractures tend to be less stable and may require fixation with wires.

Treatment of a type III injury is more complicated. The posterior cortex is disrupted with no cortical contact and the distal fragment is displaced posteriorly and proximally (by the pull of the triceps). If the fracture has medial displacement, the medial periosteal hinge is usually intact. If the fracture has lateral displacement, the lateral periosteal hinge is intact. Completely displaced fractures with no posterior intact hinge/cortex are unstable and require some form of wire fixation. Open reduction is indicated for difficult closed reduction, particularly when the brachialis muscle has button-holed though the proximal fragment.

Complications associated with this injury include neurovascular compromise and malunion. A nerve injury may be traumatic at the time of the injury or be iatrogenic during reduction and fixation. Vascular insult can lead to Volkmann ischaemic contracture of the forearm. If a vascular injury is detected early, open reduction of the fracture and a vascular repair may be necessary. Malunion of the fracture may lead to cubitus varus deformity.

KEY POINTS

- There are two types of supracondylar fracture: the extension type (most common) and the flexion type.
- A fall onto an outstretched hand may lead to an extension-type fracture whereas a fall onto the elbow produces a flexion supracondylar fracture.
- Examination of the degree of swelling and deformity as well as an assessment of neurological and vascular status of the forearm is essential.
- The nerve most commonly injured is the anterior interosseous branch of the median nerve.
- Treatment of undisplaced fractures comprises collar and cuff or an above-elbow plaster. Treatment of displaced fractures comprises manipulation under anaesthetic and stabilization with plaster and/or wires.

CASE 14: A PAINFUL THIGH FOLLOWING A VIOLENT FALL

History

A 30-year-old motorcyclist was knocked from his machine by a car and landed on the road. He complained immediately of pain in his right thigh and was unable to bear weight through his leg. He did not appear to have any other injuries. The car driver called an ambulance and the injured man has been taken to the emergency department on a stretcher.

Examination

Following a thorough assessment of head, neck, chest, pelvis and spine, it is clear that the motorcyclist has sustained an isolated injury to his femur. He has a swollen right thigh. The thigh is very tender and the patient is unable to move the leg because of pain. There are no obvious neurological or vascular deficits to the leg. The patient's breathing was noted to be fast at 30/min. Oxygen saturation is only 89 per cent on air. Radiographs are shown in Figs 14.1 and 14.2.

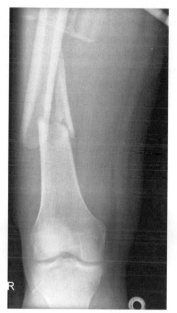

Figure 14.1

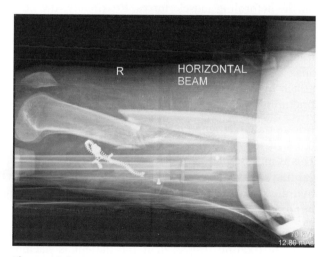

Figure 14.2

Questions

- What is the diagnosis?
- What are the mechanisms of injury?
- How would you manage this patient?

ANSWER 14

The diagnosis is a fracture of the femoral shaft. The X-rays show significant shortening and displacement.

These types of fracture are usually caused by direct, high-energy forces, and may be life-threatening. Isolated fractures can occur with repetitive stress and in the presence of metabolic bone disorders, or primary or secondary bone tumours. The area most susceptible to stress fracture is the medial junction of the proximal and middle third of the femur, which occurs as a result of the compression forces on the medial femur. Stress fractures can also occur on the lateral aspect of the femoral neck in areas of distraction and are less likely to heal non-operatively compared to compression-sided stress fractures.

One of the risks following a femoral shaft fracture is fat embolism leading to respiratory compromise – which would account for this patient's increased respiratory rate and hypoxia.

Femoral fracture patterns vary according to the mechanism of injury. The fracture depends on the direction of the force applied and the quantity of the energy absorbed. A perpendicular force results in a transverse fracture pattern, an axial force may injure the hip or knee, and rotational forces may cause spiral or oblique fracture patterns. The amount of comminution present depends on the amount of energy absorbed by the femur at the time of injury. The degree of translation, angulation and rotation depends on the deforming muscle forces. Proximally, the gluteus medius and minimus attach to the greater trochanter, resulting in abduction of the femur with fracture. The iliopsoas attaches to the lesser trochanter, resulting in internal rotation and external rotation with fractures. Distally, the large adductor muscle mass attaches medially, resulting in an apex lateral deformity with fractures. The medial and lateral heads of the gastrocnemius attach over the posterior femoral condyles, resulting in flexion deformity in distal-third fractures.

Appropriate resuscitation of the patient is necessary prior to any definitive surgery. The femur is very vascular, so fractures can result in 2–3 units of blood loss into the thigh. This is an essential part of resuscitation, particularly in elderly individuals who have less cardiac reserve. Patients should be monitored for fat embolism syndrome and kept well hydrated and oxygenated – as in this case as the man has a raised respiratory rate and hypoxia.

The majority of femoral shaft fractures are treated surgically with intramedullary nails or plate fixation. However, if the patient is haemodynamically unstable and has not been adequately resuscitated, femoral fixation should be delayed and temporized with an external fixator or skeletal traction. Plate fixation may be used when femoral fractures are associated with vascular injury that requires repair or with ipsilateral femoral neck fractures. The aim of treatment is to restore the length, alignment and rotation of the bone as soon as possible. The majority of femoral shaft fractures are united by 3–5 months.

 KEY POINTS

- Following a femoral shaft fracture, fat embolism can lead to respiratory compromise.
- Femoral shaft fractures can result in up to 2–3 units of blood loss.
- The majority of femoral shaft fractures are treated surgically with intramedullary nails or plate fixation, *following adequate resuscitation*.

CASE 15: GROIN PAIN FOLLOWING A FALL

History

A 79-year-old woman has presented to the emergency department after a fall. She has been lying on a hard floor for over 6 hours before she managed to call an ambulance. She complains of pain in the groin and inability to bear weight on the affected side. She is on warfarin for atrial fibrillation. Her mental test score is 10 out of 10. She previously walked short distances with the aid of one stick.

Examination

The affected leg has shortening and external rotation, and she is unable to actively move her hip due to the pain. A radiograph is shown in Fig. 15.1.

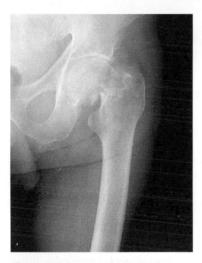

Figure 15.1

Questions

- What is the diagnosis?
- If you could not see the injury clearly on plain X-rays in a patient with pain, what investigation would you request next?
- How would you classify this injury?
- Describe the blood supply to the femoral head
- How would you manage this patient's injury?
- How would you manage a patient with an extracapsular fracture of their proximal femur?

ANSWER 15

The diagnosis is a fractured neck of femur. The leg is short, externally rotated and she is unable to bear weight, and the X-ray shows a displaced intracapsular fracture of the proximal femur.

Hip fractures are the most common reason for admission to an orthopaedic ward, usually caused by a fall by an elderly person. The average age of a person with a hip fracture is 77 years. Mortality is high: about 10 per cent of people with a hip fracture die within 1 month, and about one-third within 12 months. However, fewer than half of deaths are attributable to the fracture, reflecting the high prevalence of comorbidity. The mental status of the patient is also important: senility is associated with a three-fold increased risk of sepsis and dislocation of prosthetic replacement when compared with mentally alert patients. The one-year mortality rate in these patients is considerable, being reported as high as 50 per cent.

MRI is the investigation of choice where there is doubt about the diagnosis. If MRI is not available or not feasible, a radioisotope bone scan or repeat plain radiographs (after an interval of 24–48 hours) should be performed.

Garden's classification is the most widely accepted for grading a fractured neck of femur (see the box). The present case is stage IV.

The blood supply to the proximal end of the femur is divided into three major groups.

- The first is the extracapsular arterial ring located at the base of the femoral neck.
- The second is the ascending cervical branches of the arterial ring on the surface of the femoral neck.
- The third is the arteries of the ligamentum teres.

A large branch of the medial femoral circumflex artery forms the extracapsular arterial ring posteriorly and anteriorly by a branch from the lateral femoral circumflex artery. The ascending cervical branches ascend on the surface of the femoral neck anteriorly along the intertrochanteric line. Posteriorly, the cervical branches run under the synovial reflection towards the rim of the articular cartilage, which demarcates the femoral neck from its head. The lateral vessels are the most vulnerable to injury in femoral neck fractures.

Management of this patient should follow the national recommended guidelines. An early assessment in the emergency department or ward should include a formal assessment of the pressure sore risk, hydration and nutrition, fluid balance, pain, core body temperature, continence, coexisting medical problems, mental state, previous mobility, previous functional ability, social circumstances and whether the patient has a carer.

This patient had been lying on a hard floor for 6 hours and is deemed to be at high risk of pressure sores. She should be nursed on a large-cell alternating-pressure air mattress or comparable pressure-reducing surface. Soft-tissue surfaces should be used to protect the heel and sacrum from pressure damage. The patient should be kept warm, be provided with adequate analgesia and early assessment and correction of any fluid and electrolyte disturbances.

Ideally during the preoperative period the patient should be managed on an orthopaedic ward with orthogeriatric medical support. This patient is on warfarin; withholding warfarin combined with administration of oral or intravenous vitamin K is recommended for reversal of the anticoagulant effect of warfarin to permit earlier surgery if deemed appropriate. Where it is deemed appropriate to use it, fresh frozen plasma (FFP) should be used. The routine use of traction (either skin or skeletal) is *not* recommended prior to surgery for a hip fracture.

Infection rates can be reduced by preoperative antibiotic prophylaxis. Use of chemical or mechanical thromboprophylaxis for 28 days is recommended.

The surgical management of intracapsular fractures with undisplaced fractures should be internal fixation with hip screws. However, assessment prior to surgery should consider the patient's mobility, mental state and pre-existing bone and joint pathology. This patient has a displaced intracapsular hip fracture. If she were a young patient, closed reduction and internal fixation could be considered, to try to save the femoral head. If she were a more active individual, a total hip replacement could also have been an option. In this patient's case, a cemented hemiarthroplasty is recommended. In the presence of significant cardiorespiratory disease, an uncemented hemiarthroplasty would have been recommended.

All extracapsular fractures of the proximal femur should be treated surgically unless there are medical contraindications. A sliding hip screw is recommended except with particular fractures (e.g. reverse oblique, transverse or subtrochanteric features) where an intramedullary device may be considered as this will provide more biomechanical stability while the fracture is healing.

! **Garden's classification of femoral neck fractures**

- Stage I: Incomplete/impacted fracture; medial trabeculae of the head are tilted posterolaterally
- Stage II: Complete but undisplaced fracture; alignments of the medial trabeculae of the neck head and acetabulum are undisturbed
- Stage III: Complete, partially displaced fracture; medial trabeculae of the head are rotated medially
- Stage IV: Complete, fully displaced fracture; medial trabeculae of the head are aligned with those of the acetabulum

---

KEY POINTS

- Fractured neck of femur is the most common cause for admission to an orthopaedic ward. It carries a high mortality rate.
- Blood supply of the femoral head is critical in minimally displaced fractures.
- Displaced intracapsular fractures are treated with arthroplasty. Displaced extracapsular fractures are treated with open reduction and internal fixation.

CASE 16: A SWOLLEN PAINFUL LEG AFTER A SPORTING INCIDENT

History

A 22-year-old man was playing football when he was involved in a heavy tackle. He heard a crack and fell to the ground. He felt pain in his left leg and was unable to bear weight. The team physiotherapist and doctor were called and the man was taken on a stretcher to hospital as his pain worsened.

Examination

This footballer has some moderate swelling of the leg. It is a closed injury. On palpation of the tibia, he has extreme tenderness mid way down, and the leg also appears deformed. Distal pulses and sensation are present. Radiographs are shown in Figs 16.1 and 16.2.

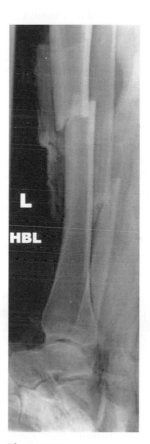

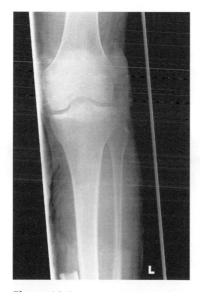

Figure 16.1   Figure 16.2

Questions

- What is the diagnosis?
- How would you classify this injury if it were instead an open fracture?
- How would you manage this injury?

ANSWER 16

The diagnosis is a fracture of the tibial shaft. The tibia is the most frequent site of a long-bone fracture in the body. Shaft fractures are often the result of high-energy trauma, but they can occur as a result of overuse causing a stress fracture. With a stress fracture, there is often a history of a recent change in activity level and the pain typically increases during weight-bearing and improves with rest.

The classification system most widely adopted for open tibial shaft fractures is Gustilo and Anderson's (see the box).

Open fractures are surgical emergencies and ideally should be taken to the operating theatre as soon as possible or put on the next available operating list. In the emergency room, an antibiotic should be administered, plus analgesia and a splint. Careful documentation of the neurovascular status should be made. Plastic surgical expertise may be required to provide soft-tissue coverage at the same time as stabilizing the fracture with either an intramedullary nail or external fixator.

These injuries carry risk of various complications, including infection (particularly with open fractures), delayed union (particularly in smokers), malunion (often the tibia will fall into varus with distal fractures and will fall into valgus with proximal fractures), and non-union (especially in the presence of significant periosteal striping and poor soft-tissue cover and significant comminution and displacement).

Most closed tibial fractures can be treated conservatively using plaster of Paris. The knee is typically flexed to 10–15 degrees and the ankle dorsiflexed to neutral. Admission to hospital may be necessary to control pain and monitor for compartment syndrome. Follow-up radiographs should initially be frequent to assess whether satisfactory reduction has been maintained. Total cast time can be up to 3 months, with initial non-weight-bearing and progressing to full weight-bearing over the period. At 6 weeks, if there is satisfactory evidence of fracture heal, the above-knee cast can be converted to a below-knee one (patella tendon-bearing Sarmiento cast).

Tibial shaft fractures treated with casting must be monitored closely with frequent radiographs to ensure that the fracture has maintained adequate alignment. Adequate callus formation generally takes 12 weeks before cast therapy can be discontinued.

In this patient, the displaced tibia fracture is unstable and should be fixed operatively. An unstable fracture is present when there is greater than 1.5 cm of shortening, more than 5 degrees of varus or valgus angulation, 10 degrees of anterior or posterior angulation, and/or greater than 50 per cent translation while the leg is in a plaster. Specific factors that contribute to instability include comminution, fibular fracture and very proximal, segmental or distal fracture. Intramedullary nailing and external fixation have replaced fracture plating because they are associated with reduced infection rates, and damage to local soft tissues. In the majority, tibial nails are not removed and may remain in the patient indefinitely. If they cause specific problems such as anterior knee pain and the locking screws are prominent, then either the screws alone, and in some cases the nail as well, can be removed once the fracture has united.

> **!** | **Gustilo and Anderson's grading of tibial shaft fractures**
>
> - Type I: Wound remains clean and is less than 1 cm in length
> - Type II: Wound is longer than 1 cm and does not have extensive soft-tissue damage
> - Type IIIa: Wound is associated with extensive soft-tissue damage, usually larger than 1 cm with periosteal coverage
> - Type IIIb: Fracture has periosteal stripping that must be covered (nearly always require soft-tissue flap coverage)
> - Type IIIc: Fracture is associated with vascular injury that requires repair

KEY POINTS

- Tibial shaft fractures are often the result of high-energy trauma but can also occur as a result of overuse.
- Look for open wounds at the fracture site, neurovascular compromise, and elevated compartment pressure.
- Open fractures are surgical emergencies and ideally should be taken to the operating theatre as soon as possible or put on the next available operating list.
- Plastic surgical expertise may be required to provide soft-tissue coverage.
- Most closed tibial fractures can be treated conservatively using plaster of Paris. Fractures that are unstable should be fixed operatively.

CASE 17: A PAINFUL AND SWOLLEN KNEE FOLLOWING AN ACCIDENT

History
A 45-year-old man was crossing a road when he was hit by a car at the level of the vehicle's bumper. The point of impact was the lateral aspect of his left knee. He developed swelling of his knee immediately. He was unable to bear weight. An ambulance took him to the emergency department.

Examination
This man has an isolated injury to his left knee. The knee is swollen and, on palpation, he has tenderness in his lateral joint line, and pain when applying valgus stress to his knee. He is unable to move his knee because of the pain. He has no neurovascular deficit and no evidence of compartment syndrome. Radiographs are shown in Figs 17.1 and 17.2.

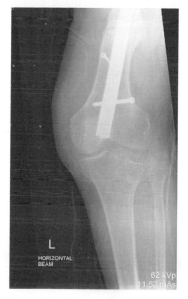

Figure 17.1

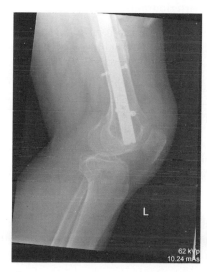

Figure 17.2

Questions
- What is the diagnosis?
- Describe how you would assess this injury clinically and radiologically.
- Describe the classification system for this type of injury and the associated injuries.
- Describe the principles of management.

ANSWER 17

The diagnosis is a fracture of the tibial plateau. This fracture disrupts the articular surface of the proximal tibia and causes a haemarthosis and immediate swelling of the knee. The peak incidence occurs in men in their fourth decade and in women in their seventh decade. The increased incidence of tibial plateau fractures in older women is predominantly due to osteoporosis and they tend to be depression type fractures. Tibial plateau fractures in younger patients are commonly the result of high-energy injuries and tend to be splitting-type fractures.

Knowing the mechanism of injury is important because it may aid in determining whether the injury was high- or low-velocity. The presence of a haemarthrosis should be noted. Compare the knees to assess for any deformity. Gentle stress testing can be performed with the leg in extension to evaluate the stability of the ligaments. With a lateral impact injury the medial collateral ligament may have been injured. Leg compartments should be assessed for any evidence of a compartment syndrome. A careful neurological examination should be performed particularly to exclude injury to the peroneal nerve. Any concern for possible vascular injury to the popliteal artery should be aggressively pursued with an arteriogram.

Following the clinical examination, initial anteroposterior and lateral and oblique radiographs should be obtained. When assessing the lateral radiograph, remember the lateral plateau is convex and the medial plateau is concave. CT scans can assist in determining the extent and location of fracture lines and depressed fragments.

There are a number of classification systems, the most widely adopted being the Schatzker classification. There are six types.

- Type I is a wedge fracture of the lateral tibial plateau and is most commonly seen in younger patients.
- Type II is a split fracture associated with depression of the lateral plateau. The underlying bone may be osteoporotic. The mechanism of injury is typically a combination of valgus stress and axial compression force. Look out for associated injuries such as a fracture of the fibular head and neck, ligamentous injuries, particularly the medial collateral ligament, and avulsion of bone from the medial femoral condyle.
- Type III is a pure depression fracture of the lateral tibial plateau. The flexion angle of the knee at injury determines the depth of depression.
- Type IV is a fracture of the medial tibial plateau and carries the worst prognosis of all the tibial plateau fractures. There are two type IV injuries. The low-energy fracture in elderly patients with osteoporotic bone can lead to significant compression. The high-energy fractures typically occur in younger patients and can be associated with intercondylar eminence fracture, lateral ligament rupture and/or peroneal nerve traction injury.
- Type V is a fracture of both the medial and lateral tibial condyles. This injury occurs with an axial force while the knee is in extension. Because these are high-energy injuries, they may be associated with soft-tissue injuries including peripheral meniscal detachment, anterior cruciate ligament avulsions, neurovascular injuries and knee dislocation, thereby adding to the knee instability and compartment syndrome.
- Type VI is a complex, bicondylar fracture in which the condylar fragments are separate from the diaphysis. This pattern of injury is the result of high-energy trauma. This injury is also associated with partial or complete ruptures and/or meniscal tears.

Fracture displacement ranging up to 5 mm can be treated conservatively; however, a depressed fragment greater than 5 mm should be considered for elevation and bone grafting. The goals of tibial plateau fracture treatment are to restore joint stability, alignment, and articular congruity while preserving full range of motion. Internal fixation techniques include ligamentotaxis, percutaneous fixation, and antiglide techniques. When extensive comminution and damaged soft tissues prohibit the use of internal fixation, circular external fixators are an excellent fallback option for management.

 KEY POINTS

- Tibial plateau fractures in older women are predominantly due to osteoporosis and tend to be depression-type fractures. In younger patients they are commonly the result of high-energy injuries and tend to be splitting-type fractures.
- Anteroposterior and lateral and oblique radiographs should be obtained. CT scans can assist in determining the extent and location of fracture lines and depressed fragments.
- Fracture displacement up to 5 mm can be treated conservatively.
- The goals of treatment are to restore joint stability, alignment, and articular congruity while preserving full range of motion.

CASE 18: A CRUSHED LEG

History

A 25-year-old fire-fighter had been tackling a warehouse fire. During the aftermath, some of the building collapsed and his leg was crushed by a slab of concrete. It took 2 hours to release him and take him to hospital.

Examination

This young man's right leg shows extensive bruising and swelling, as well as dust from the concrete. On palpation, the right calf is very tense anteriorly and posteriorly. The patient also complains of intense pain on passive stretching of his toes. He reports some altered sensation in the right foot compared to the left. His foot pulses are, however, present. The radiograph shows a transverse fracture through the mid shaft of the tibia. The man's pain is not being relieved with morphine despite increasing doses.

Questions

- What is the diagnosis?
- What are the causes of this condition?
- Who is at risk of this diagnosis?
- How would you further examine, investigate and manage this patient?

ANSWER 18

Compartment syndrome is the diagnosis, given the history of a crushing injury, underlying tibial shaft fracture, tense compartment of the leg and pain on passive stretching. This condition is an orthopaedic emergency and can be limb- and life-threatening.

Compartment syndrome occurs when perfusion pressure falls below tissue pressure in a closed fascial compartment and results in microvascular compromise. At this point, blood flow through the capillaries stops. In the absence of flow, oxygen delivery stops. Hypoxic injury causes cells to release vasoactive substances (e.g. histamine, serotonin), which increase endothelial permeability. Capillaries allow continued fluid loss, which increases tissue pressure and advances injury. Nerve conduction slows, tissue pH falls due to anaerobic metabolism, surrounding tissue suffers further damage, and muscle tissue suffers necrosis, releasing myoglobin. In untreated cases the syndrome can lead to permanent functional impairment, renal failure secondary to rhabdomyolysis, and death.

Patients at risk of compartment syndrome include those with high-velocity injuries, long-bone fractures, high-energy trauma, penetrating injuries such as gunshot wounds and stabbing, and crush injuries, as well as patients on anticoagulants with trauma.

The patient usually complains of severe pain that is out of proportion to the injury. An assessment of the affected limb may reveal swelling which feels tense, or hard compartments. Pain on passive range of movement of fingers or toes of the affected limb is a typical feature. Late signs comprise pallor, paralysis, paraesthesia and a pulseless limb. Sensory nerves begin to lose conductive ability, followed by motor nerves. Some nerves may reveal effects of increasing pressure before others. For example, in the anterior compartment of the lower leg the deep peroneal nerve is quickly affected, and sensation in the web space between the first two toes may be lost.

The development of a compartment syndrome depends on compartment pressure as well as systemic blood pressure. The diastolic blood pressure minus the compartment pressure should be less than 30 mmHg. A formal assessment of the compartment pressure should be performed and pressures greater than 30 mmHg are generally agreed to require intervention.

In the present case, all the dressings and casts should be removed down to skin as it has been shown that splitting of the underlying dressings reduces the pressure by a further 15 per cent, while complete removal of casts leads to a further reduction of 15 per cent. The limb should be kept at the level of the heart rather than elevated, to maximize tissue perfusion. Supplementary oxygen slightly increases the partial pressure of oxygen to the tissues. Hypovolaemia can worsen ischaemia, and intravenous hydration should be administered.

This patient needs to go to theatre and have stabilization of his fracture. Fasciotomy is the definitive treatment for compartment syndrome. The purpose of fasciotomy is to achieve prompt and adequate decompression so as to restore the tissue perfusion. The surgeon should be familiar with the visual recognition of necrotic tissue because thorough debridement reduces the potential of infection and improves the chances of tissue recovery. Regardless of the approach used, all compartments of the leg must be thoroughly decompressed. A delay in surgery could lead to ischaemic contractures or even amputation.

KEY POINTS

- Compartment syndrome is an orthopaedic emergency. Perfusion pressure falls below tissue pressure in a closed fascial compartment.
- Risk situations include high-energy trauma and crush injuries.
- The patient usually complains of severe pain that is out of proportion to the obvious injury.
- Compartment pressure greater than 30 mmHg requires intervention. Fasciotomy is the definitive treatment.

CASE 19: A PAINFUL FOOT FOLLOWING A TRAFFIC INCIDENT

History

A 45-year-old builder was driving to work when a cyclist swerved in front of him. He swerved but crashed the van despite some forceful braking. The van was crushed and the brake pedal had to be cut to free his foot. He reported that his foot was extremely painful and he was taken to hospital.

Examination

The builder says that he has pain in his hind foot only. On inspection he has a closed injury with significant midfoot swelling. He has no neurovascular deficit. He had palpable tenderness just proximal to his midfoot. Radiographs are shown in Figs 19.1 and 19.2.

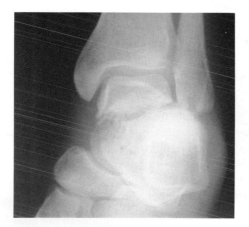

Figure 19.1   Figure 19.2

Questions

- What is the diagnosis?
- What other injuries are associated with this injury?
- Describe the blood supply to the talus.
- What are possible complications of this injury?

WER 19

The diagnosis is a talus fracture. The lateral X-ray shows a displaced fracture through the talar neck. The classification of talar neck fractures was described by Hawkins in 1970.

- With type I injuries, the talar neck fracture remains undisplaced.
- With type II injuries, the talar neck fracture is displaced and the subtalar joint is subluxated or dislocated. (In the present case the talar neck is fractured but the subtalar joint is not dislocated.)
- With type III injuries, the talar neck fracture is displaced and the body of the talus is dislocated from both the subtalar and ankle joints. The body is usually extruded posteromedially to rest between the Achilles tendon and the posterior surface of the tibia.
- With type IV injuries, a displaced talar neck fracture is associated with dislocation of the talar body from both the subtalar and ankle joints, and dislocation of the talar head from the talonavicular joint.

Hawkins's sign is the appearance of a zone of osteopenia or lucency under the subchondral bone of the talar dome.

Associated injuries are common, and frequently include the medial malleous and lumbar spine fractures.

The middle portion of the talar body receives its blood supply from the tarsal canal artery, which consistently arises 2 cm below the ankle from the posterior tibial artery. About 5 mm from its origin the tarsal canal artery gives off a deltoid branch, which supplies the medial quarter of the talar body. The dorsalis pedis and peroneal arteries have branches which anastomose to form the tarsal sinus artery. The tarsal sinus artery provides blood to the lateral aspect of the talar body and the majority of the talar head.

With type I fractures the intraosseous vessels coursing from distal to proximal in the talar neck are disrupted, so the avascular necrosis (AVN) rate of the talar body ranges from 0 to 10 per cent. With type II fractures, the intraosseous blood supply and the vessels coursing inferiorly from the tarsal sinus artery are damaged (likely in the present case). The AVN rate is 20–50 per cent. With type III fractures, the AVN rate ranges from 50 to 100 per cent, as the intraosseous, tarsal sinus, tarsal canal and deltoid vessels are all injured. With type IV fractures, the risk of AVN of the talar body approaches 100 per cent and damage to the blood supply to the talar head occurs as well.

 KEY POINTS

- Talus fractures occur with forced dorsiflexion injury.
- The talus has a tenuous blood supply.
- Associated injuries are common, and frequently include the medial malleolus and lumbar spine fractures.
- Risk of avascular necrosis depends on the degree of displacement and ranges from 10 to 100 per cent.
- Hawkins's sign is the appearance of a zone of osteopenia or lucency under the subchondral bone of the talar dome.

CASE 20: A HINDFOOT INJURY FOLLOWING A FALL FROM HEIGHT

History

A 30-year-old roofer was repairing tiles when he fell from a ladder. The fall was about 3 metres. He landed on his feet, taking most of the impact on one of his heels. At the time of the incident he complained of severe isolated pain in his hindfoot only. He has reported no symptoms of pain in his lumbar spine.

Examination

This man has marked swelling in his hindfoot associated with bruising compared to the other side. On palpation, he has no tenderness in his lateral or medial malleolus, but he has severe pain in his hindfoot. He is reluctant to move his ankle but is able to do so fully. He has no evidence of any neurological or vascular deficits in his foot, with a good dorsalis pedis and posterior tibialis pulse. Assessment of his gait shows that he is unable to bear weight on the injured foot. A radiograph is shown in Fig. 20.1.

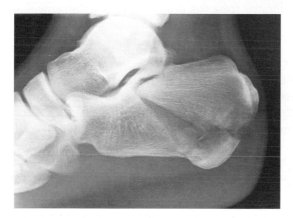

Figure 20.1

Questions

- What is the diagnosis?
- What other injuries can be associated with this injury?
- What are the radiological features of this injury?
- How would you manage this patient?

ANSWER 20

The diagnosis is a calcaneum fracture. The most common situation leading to calcaneal fracture is a young adult who falls from a height and lands on his or her feet. Fractures of the os calcis are the most common tarsal fractures.

Patients often sustain occult injuries to their lumbar or cervical spine, and the proximal femur. A thorough clinical and radiological investigation of the spine area is mandatory in patients with calcaneal fracture.

X-rays should include anteroposterior, lateral, oblique, axial and Broden views. The AP radiograph allows assessment of any calcaneocuboid joint involvement, talonavicular subluxation, and lateral wall widening. AP views of the ankle are used to assess for any subfibular impingement in the presence of lateral displacement of the lateral wall of the calcaneus.

Lateral radiographs show the fracture line through the calcaneum. The lateral radiographs of the foot are used to evaluate the Bohler angle. This angle is defined by two intersecting lines. One line is drawn from the anterior process of the calcaneus to the peak of the posterior articular surface. The second is drawn from the peak of the posterior articular surface to the peak of the posterior tuberosity. The angle is normally between 25 and 40 degrees. In severe fractures with subtalar joint involvement, this angle may decrease or become negative.

Oblique views show the degree of displacement of the primary fracture line and the lesser facets. Axial views help show the primary fracture line, any varus malpositioning, posterior facet step-off, lateral-wall displacement, and fibular abutment. Broden views of the foot are obtained by internally rotating the leg 45 degrees with the ankle in neutral position. The beam may then be directed toward the lateral malleolus to evaluate the posterior facet. CT scans show the degree of comminution of the posterior facet of the calcaneum and also help with classification and planning of treatment.

Treatment goals of operative modalities include restoration of the heel height and length, realignment of the posterior facet of the subtalar joint, and restoration of the mechanical axis of the hindfoot either conservatively with plaster or open reduction and internal fixation with plate and screws.

 KEY POINTS

- Fractures of the os calcis are the most common tarsal fractures.
- Exclude any concomitant spinal injury.
- CT scans aid in assessing the classification and planning treatment.
- Conservative management in a cast is used for stable and undisplaced fractures. Consider open reduction and internal fixation for displaced and unstable fractures.

CASE 21: CURVATURE OF THE SPINE

History

A 14-year-old boy has been taken to his general practitioner by his parents, who noticed that their son was developing a spine deformity. His mother says that he recently underwent a growth spurt and his spine curvature has increased significantly with this spurt. The boy complains of no pain in his spine. Despite the lack of pain, the father is concerned.

Examination

This boy has a convex right thoracic curve, as shown in Fig. 21.1. The height of the right shoulder is higher than the left and there is a prominent shoulder blade, with asymmetrical waist creases and heights of the iliac crests. On bending forward a rib hump prominence can be observed in the thoracic region of the spine. Neurological examination of all the limbs is normal. Radiographs are shown in Fig. 21.2.

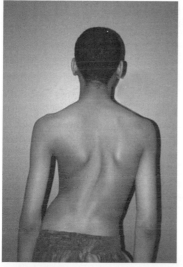

Figure 21.1

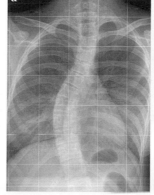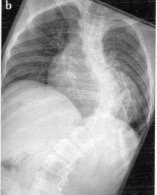

Figure 21.2

Questions

- What is the diagnosis?
- What types of this condition are most commonly seen?
- What are the most effective clinical examination screening tools for this condition?
- What studies should be performed in the congenital form of this condition?

ANSWER 21

This young boy has a diagnosis of idiopathic scoliosis due to the curvature of his spine. This is the most common spinal deformity. The prevalence of scoliosis is highest in patients aged 12–14 years. For a spinal deformity to be classified as scoliosis, both lateral (coronal plane) curvature and rotation (transverse plane) must be present – as in this case. Lateral (coronal) curvatures of less than 10 degrees are generally not referred to as scoliosis. The three types of idiopathic scoliosis are infantile (birth to 3 years), juvenile (3 years to puberty) and adolescent (at or just after puberty).

The types of this condition most commonly seen are congenital, neuromuscular and non-structural. Scoliosis is also seen in other disease processes such as neurofibromatosis, mesenchymal disease (Marfan syndrome, Ehlers–Danlos syndrome), tumours, traumatic spinal injuries, infections, spondylolisthesis and degenerative conditions.

Adam's forward-bending test (in conjunction with the use of a scoliometer) has been found to be an effective screening tool. Physical examination should include a baseline assessment of posture and body contour. Shoulder asymmetry and protruding scapulae are common. In the most common curve pattern (right thoracic), the right shoulder is consistently rotated forward and the medial border of the right scapula protrudes posteriorly.

All patients should undergo a full neurological examination, including assessment of upper and lower limb reflexes as well as the abdominal reflexes. Look for the presence or absence of hamstring tightness, and screening should be performed for ataxia and/or poor balance or proprioception (the Romberg test). One or two different methods of measuring leg length will prove valuable, as a significant percentage of patients presenting with scoliosis have limb-length discrepancy. Palpation of the spine is usually painless.

A string test often helps to confirm the diagnosis. A string fitted with a small weight is held over the C7 spinous process and allowed to drop straight down. It should normally fall in the midline of the gluteal natal cleft. In the presence of uncompensated scoliosis, the string will fall on one side of the natal cleft. In balanced or compensated scoliosis, the string will fall in the midline. AP and lateral X-rays of the spine assess the deformity. To measure the degree of curvature, the Cobb's angle and the rib vertebral angle difference of Mehta are used.

Genitourinary anomalies and intraspinal anomalies are associated with congenital scoliosis. An ultrasound examination of the retroperitoneum may reveal anomalies of the kidneys and genitourinary system. MRI should be undertaken in the initial evaluation of congenital scoliosis, even in the absence of clinical findings.

 KEY POINTS

- The prevalence of scoliosis is highest in patients aged 12–14 years.
- Both lateral (coronal plane) curvature and rotation (transverse plane) must be present. The most common curve pattern is right thoracic.
- Adam's forward-bending test is an effective screening tool. Shoulder asymmetry and protruding scapulae are common. To measure the degree of curvature, the Cobb's angle and the rib vertebral angle difference of Mehta are used.
- MRI should be undertaken in the initial evaluation of congenital scoliosis.
- Treatment options for idiopathic scoliosis may be observation, orthosis or operative intervention.

CASE 22: SEVERE LOW BACK PAIN

History

A 53-year-old woman developed severe back pain while shopping. She lifted heavy bags into her car and experienced worsening back pain as she drove home. It was difficult for her to find a comfortable position. Later in the day she noticed that the pain was now radiating down the back of both legs. She had no sensation in her buttocks and was having episodes of urinary incontinence. She was extremely anxious about the condition, so her husband took her to the emergency department, where she needed assistance to get into the building for assessment.

Questions

- What is the diagnosis?
- What causes this condition?
- How would you investigate it?
- How would you manage this patient?

ANSWER 22

The diagnosis is cauda equina syndrome and is an orthopaedic emergency. The condition is characterized by the red-flag signs comprising low back pain, unilateral or bilateral sciatica, saddle anaesthesia with sacral sparing, and bladder and bowel dysfunctions. Urinary retention is the most consistent finding. Initially the patient may report difficulty starting or stopping a stream of urine, and this may be followed by frank incontinence, first of urine and then stool.

Rectal examination often reveals poor anal tone. The urinary incontinence is secondary to overflow. There may be a variable lower extremity motor and sensory loss depending on the affected nerve roots. The reflexes may be present, but they are typically reduced or absent.

The cauda eqina is below the level of the conus medullaris. Here the spinal canal is filled with the cauda equina, which consists of motor and sensory nerve roots. Lesions can compress the cauda equina nerve roots. Examples are large central disc prolapse, primary or secondary metastatic disease to the spine, epidural abscess or haematoma, and trauma. It may also be the result of surgical morbidity.

MRI is the investigation of choice. The scan also assists in the diagnosis of the primary problem.

Urgent spinal orthopaedic or neurosurgical consultation is essential, with transfer to a unit capable of undertaking any definitive surgery considered necessary. In the long term, residual weakness, incontinence, impotence and/or sensory abnormalities are potential problems if therapy is delayed. The early use of steroids is widely debated. The prognosis improves if a definitive cause is identified and appropriate surgical spinal decompression occurs early. Late surgical decompression produces varying results and is often associated with a poorer outcome.

 KEY POINTS

- Cauda equina syndrome is an orthopaedic emergency.
- Red-flag signs are low back pain, unilateral or bilateral sciatica, saddle anaesthesia with sacral sparing, and bladder and bowel dysfunctions.
- Urgent spinal orthopaedic or neurosurgical consult is essential.

CASE 23: A CLICKY HIP IN A TODDLER

History

A 4-year-old first-born girl has been taken by her parents to a paediatric outpatient clinic because they are concerned about their daughter's hips clicking, although they believe there is no associated pain. The mother reports having the same problem when she was a child and vaguely recalls her mother saying that she had to be put into a plaster. Like her mother, the baby was delivered via the breech position. During the gestation, the mother was diagnosed with oligohydramnios.

Examination

The child has no obvious distress or pain. On inspection of her hips, she has evidence of asymmetrical skin creases. Movement of the right hip leads to a reproducible clunking. A radiograph and clinical picture are shown in Figs 23.1 and 23.2.

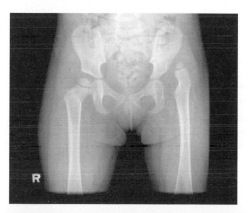

Figure 23.1

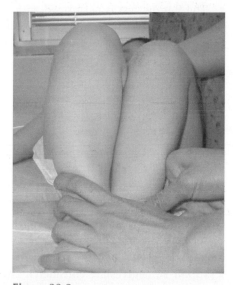

Figure 23.2

Questions

- What is the diagnosis?
- What are the risk factors for this condition?
- What are the clinical tests used to help diagnosis?
- What further radiology would you use to investigate this hip?
- How would you manage this patient?

ANSWER 23

The diagnosis is developmental dysplasia of the hips (DDH). It is characterized by asymmetrical skin creases, clunking hip, leg length discrepancy and radiographic signs. DDH is defined as abnormal growth of the hip. Affected individuals can have a hip condition ranging from asymptomatic with only subtle radiographic signs, to mild instability, to frank dislocation(s) with acetabular abnormality.

The risk factors are female sex, breech presentation at birth, primiparous baby, high birthweight, family history, multiple pregnancy and oligohydramnios.

Ortolani and Barlow tests help detect unstable hips in infancy.

- The Ortolani test is performed by placing the thumb over the inner thigh and the index finger on the greater trochanter. The hip is abducted and gentle pressure is placed over the greater trochanter. A clunk is felt when the hip is reduced. Ortolani postulated that a positive test was associated with reduction of the hip into the acetabulum.
- The Barlow test is performed with the hips in an adducted position and slight gentle posterior pressure applied to the hips. A clunk should be felt as the hip subluxes out of the acetabulum.

The Galeazzi sign can be used to detect unilateral hip dislocation. This is performed with the patient lying supine and the hips and knees flexed. Examination should demonstrate that one leg appears shorter than the other. Although this is usually due to hip dislocation, it is important to realize that any limb length discrepancy will result in a positive Galeazzi sign. Limited abduction of the affected hip is also a common finding with unilateral DDH.

Additional physical examination findings for late dislocation include asymmetry of the gluteal thigh or labral skin folds. Associated abnormalities include metatarsus adductus and torticollis. Bilateral dislocation of the hip can be quite difficult to diagnose and often manifests as a waddling gait with hyperlordosis.

Ultrasound plays an important role in both the diagnosis and treatment of DDH. The alpha angle is used to measure the acetabular concavity. A normal alpha angle is 60 degrees. Angles of 50–60 degrees are considered immature and require follow-up. Angles less than 50 degrees are considered abnormal.

Early diagnosis aids in the successful treatment of DDH. The principal aim is to get the femoral head into the acetabulum to allow for normal development of the hip joint. A Pavlik harness is the treatment of choice for neonates with hip instability. Excessive hip flexion can lead to femoral nerve compression and inferior dislocations. Excessive abduction should be avoided because of concern regarding the development of avascular necrosis of the femoral head.

Infants at 6–24 months can be managed following an assessment of whether the hip is reducible under anaesthesia and arthrography. If the hip is reducible and contained in the hip joint, a hip spica is the treatment of choice. The cast is typically worn for 6–12 weeks and, if the hip is found to be stable, the patient is then placed in an abduction brace.

Open reduction is the treatment of choice for a child presenting older than 2 years of age, or for a younger child after failed closed reduction. With infants older than 3 years (as in the present case), femoral shortening is performed instead of traction, with additional varus osteotomy to the proximal femur, if necessary. Infants older than 4 years with residual acetabular dysplasia should be treated with an acetabular osteotomy procedure. Early degenerative osteoarthritis is likely to occur unless the hip is reduced.

KEY POINTS

- DDH is defined as abnormal growth of the hip.
- Ortolani and Barlow tests help detect unstable hips in infancy.
- Ultrasound can be used to measure the alpha angle.
- Treatment options depend on the age at diagnosis.

CASE 24: HIP AND THIGH PAIN IN A 7-YEAR-OLD BOY

History

A 7-year-old boy told his parents that he was experiencing left hip pain referred to the thigh. This pain had been present for 4 weeks and was mild and intermittent. There was no memory of recent trauma or infection. The boy was taken to his general practitioner to find out why this pain had not resolved itself.

Examination

This boy is apyrexial. Examination of his gait reveals a limp. Assessment of leg length reveals 5 mm of leg length discrepancy. Movements of the hip reveal loss of internal rotation and abduction. An initial blood test reveals a normal white cell count (WCC). A radiograph is shown in Fig. 24.1.

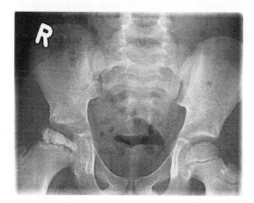

Figure 24.1

Questions
- What is the diagnosis?
- Describe the relevant X-ray features.
- How would you manage this condition?

ANSWER 24

The diagnosis is Legg–Calvé–Perthes disease (LCPD) which is the name given to idiopathic osteonecrosis of the capital femoral epiphysis of the femoral head. The leg length discrepancy can be accounted for by the collapse of the femoral head. The differential diagnosis would be septic arthritis; however, the white cell count is normal and the patient does not have a pyrexia, so that diagnosis is unlikely. Other diagnoses to consider include septic hip, transient synovitis, lymphoma, spondyloepiphyseal dysplasia, metaphyseal dysplasia, and slipped femoral capital epiphysis.

The aetiology of LCPD is unclear. The capital femoral epiphysis is always involved. In 15–20 per cent of patients with the disease, involvement is bilateral. Males are affected four to five times more often than females. LCPD is most commonly seen in individuals aged 4–8 years.

Plain X-rays of the hips and frog-leg lateral views of the affected hip are helpful in establishing the diagnosis. There are a number of classification systems, but there is no agreement as to the best. In essence, five radiographic stages can be seen by plain X-ray. Initially there is cessation of growth at the capital femoral epiphysis, with smaller femoral head epiphysis and widening of articular space on the affected side. This is followed by subchondral fracture; linear radiolucency within the femoral head epiphysis, resorption of bone as can be seen in the radiograph, re-ossification of new bone, and finally the healed stage.

Adjunct imaging comprises a technetium-99 bone scan, or MRI which is helpful in delineating avascular changes before they are evident on plain radiographs. Dynamic arthrography is helpful in assessing sphericity of the femoral head and its relationship to the acetabulum.

The goal of treatment is to avoid severe degenerative arthritis in the long term. The aim of initial treatment in this case is to relieve weight-bearing, contain the femoral epiphysis within the acetabulum, while maintaining a range of movement. Maintaining the femoral head and acetabular relationship may require the use of a brace or cast. Once the healing phase has been entered, follow-up can be every 6 months. Long-term follow-up is required to assess the final outcome and monitor for any secondary degenerative changes. In patients who fail to maintain satisfactory congruency, surgical realignment of the acetabulum and/or the proximal femur may be required.

The younger the age of onset, the more favourable the prognosis. Children older than 8–10 years tend to have a higher risk of developing osteoarthritis, typically in their fourth or fifth decade of life.

 KEY POINTS

- Legg–Calvé–Perthes disease presents most commonly at ages 4–8 years.
- Features are a smaller femoral head epiphysis, widening of articular space on the affected side, subchondral fracture, linear radiolucency within the femoral head epiphysis, resorption of bone, and re-ossification of new bone.
- Treatment involves relieving weight-bearing, containing the femoral epiphysis within the acetabulum and maintaining range of movement.
- The younger the age of onset, the more favourable the prognosis. There is a risk of developing osteoarthritis later in life.

CASE 25: A PAINFUL HIP IN AN ADOLESCENT

History

A 12-year-old overweight boy regularly walked to school. Over a period of three days he developed groin pain which now limits him. The pain is getting worse and he told his parents that it is also radiating down to his knee. He has attended the emergency department.

Examination

This boy has no obvious deformity of the affected limb. He also has no palpable tenderness. Assessment of the movement of the right hip reveals that during flexion the hip moves into external rotation as well. Radiographs are shown in Figs 25.1 and 25.2.

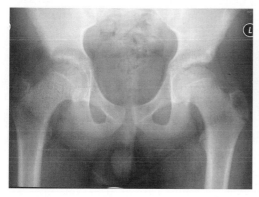

Figure 25.1

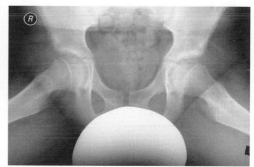

Figure 25.2

Questions

- What is the diagnosis?
- Who is at risk of developing this condition?
- Describe the radiological findings.

ANSWER 25

The diagnosis is a slipped upper femoral epiphysis (SUFE). There is a posteroinferior displacement of the proximal femoral epiphysis. This is typical in this age group. The slip occurs between the proliferative and hypertrophic zones of the growth plate. The patient can present with knee pain referred from the hip via the obturator nerve. Patients often hold the affected hip in the passive external rotation position. Flexion of the hip may lead to external rotation with minimal internal rotation – as in this case. The patient may or may not be able to bear weight. The clinical presentation may be classified as acute, chronic or acute-on-chronic. Symptoms such as hip or knee pain, limp and decreased range of motion for under 3 weeks are classified as acute – as in this case. Symptoms for longer than 3 weeks are deemed chronic. Symptoms of greater than 3 weeks' duration but presenting with an acute exacerbation of pain, limp, inability to bear weight or decreased range of motion – with or without an associated traumatic episode – are described as acute-on-chronic.

The incidence in boys is higher than in girls. SCFE typically presents between the ages of 10 and 16 years. In general, about 20 per cent of patients have bilateral involvement at the time of presentation. Obesity is a risk factor because it places more shear forces around the proximal growth plate in the hip at risk. In patients younger than 10 years, SCFE is associated with metabolic endocrine disorders (e.g. hypothyroidism, panhypopituitarism, hypogonadism, renal osteodystrophy, growth hormone abnormalities).

Anteroposterior and frog–lateral radiographs of the pelvis/hips should be obtained. Assess for any head displacement of the femoral neck, particularly posterior and inferior, as can be seen in this case on the frog–lateral X-ray view. In a mild case of SUFE, one may see widening and lack of definition of the physeal plate. Klein's line, drawn along the superior edge of the femoral neck, may not intersect with the femoral head (Trethowan's sign) – as in this case. There may be metaphyseal blanching, due to increased X-ray absorption caused by superimposition of the head behind the metaphysis. Bony changes of the femoral neck and head may be indicative of chronic history of symptoms. Chronic cases may show new bone formation on the posterior/inferior part of the femoral neck. Over time, the superior edge of the metaphysis becomes blunted and round owing to erosion caused by abutment against the acetabular labrum or acetabular edge.

 KEY POINTS

- In SUFE there is posteroinferior displacement of the proximal femoral epiphysis. Flexion of the hip may lead to external rotation with minimal internal rotation.
- SUFE is classified as acute, chronic or acute-on-chronic.
- It presents between the ages of 10 and 16 years.
- Obesity and metabolic endocrine disorders are risk factors.
- Risks include avascular necrosis.

CASE 26: GROIN AND BUTTOCK PAIN IN AN ELDERLY MAN

History

An 80-year-old man presents with progressively worsening pain in his left groin and buttock radiating to the knee with no pins and needles. There is no history of pre-existing trauma or disease in that hip. He complains of pain made worse on walking and has difficulty in putting on shoes and tying shoe laces. He obtains only partial relief of the symptoms with analgesia and rest.

Examination

The patient walks with an antalgic gait. He has a fixed flexion deformity of 10 degrees. His range of motion in the left hip is restricted and painful in all directions. There is no neurovascular deficit in the leg. Radiographs of his hip are shown in Figs 26.1 and 26.2.

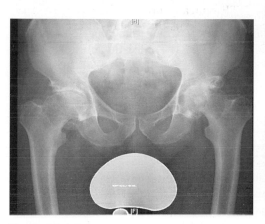

Figure 26.1   Figure 26.2

Questions

• What is the differential diagnosis?
• What other causes can predispose to this condition?
• Describe the four radiological signs in the right hip.
• What are the management options for this patient?

ANSWER 26

This elderly patient has insidious onset and deteriorating pain in his right hip. The pain is located in the groin and buttock and radiates to the knee.

The initial approach is to determine that the hip pain is actually arising from the hip. In most cases the pathology from the hip joint results in groin pain that radiates to the thigh and knee. Patients with hip pathology can sometimes present with knee pain without any groin or thigh symptoms. Pain in the sacroiliac area or below the knee is usually due to pathologies outside the hip joint. The absence of neurological symptoms in this case also indicates that the pain is likely to be mechanical in nature and arising from the hip. The history indicates that he has stiffness in the affected joint, which is causing difficulty in flexing the hip in order to put on shoes and socks. The most common cause of these signs and symptoms is primary osteoarthritis of the hip joint.

In this case there has been no preceding history of trauma, so it is likely to be primary rather than secondary osteoarthritis. Clinical signs on examination may include an antalgic gait, positive Trendelenburg sign, unequal leg length, muscle wasting, and a restriction of hip joint movements. In longstanding cases, patients may develop a flexion adduction external rotation deformity in the affected leg. The fixed flexion deformity is elicited by Thomas' test. Patients may have apparent or real shortening of the affected leg with or without a pelvic tilt.

Osteoarthritis most commonly affects middle-aged and elderly patients. Any synovial joint can develop osteoarthritis. This condition can lead to degeneration of articular cartilage and is often associated with stiffness. Osteoarthritis of the hip typically presents with a history of pain in the buttock, groin, thigh and knee.

The most common cause of osteoarthritis is idiopathic. Genetic factors play a strong role in the development of primary osteoarthritis. If there is a predisposing condition that leads to destruction of the hip joint cartilage, it is called secondary osteoarthritis. Though the clinical features of secondary osteoarthritis are similar to its primary counterpart, they tend to affect younger patients. The common causes of secondary arthritis in the hip joint include:

- developmental dysplasia of the hip
- septic arthritis of the hip
- Perthes' disease
- slipped capital femoral epiphysis
- rheumatoid arthritis
- seronegative arthropathy
- trauma
- crystal arthropathy
- avascular necrosis of the femoral head.

The principal radiological investigation to evaluate osteoarthritis of the hip is an antero-posterior standing hip X-ray and lateral view of the affected hip. The four classical radiological signs of osteoarthritis are (mnemonic LOSS):

- (L)oss of joint space
- (O)steophytes (bony spurs)
- (S)ubchondral cysts on acetabular and femoral sides
- (S)ubchondral sclerosis on acetabular and femoral sides.

In severe cases, deformity or flattening of the femoral head can be seen.

The management of osteoarthritis is conservative initially, including patient education and modification of lifestyle, regular analgesia, possibly non-steroidal anti-inflammatory drugs (NSAIDS), the use of a walking stick on the contralateral side, weight reduction, and physiotherapy.

When conservative measures fail to improve or alleviate the symptoms and the individual's sleep and quality of life are affected, surgery should be considered.

- Arthroplasty (total hip replacement) is now the treatment of choice in patients with osteoarthritis of the hip. The principal benefits are pain relief, improved mobility and correction of deformity. The risks include infection, dislocation, loosening of the joint, leg vein thrombosis, periprosthetic fracture, leg length discrepancy and neurovascular injury
- Osteotomy of the proximal femur and/or acetabulum is indicated less commomly in younger individuals with early arthritis and a good range of movement. The osteotomy aims to optimize the alignment of the hip joint to provide symptomatic relief.
- Arthrodesis is indicated in rare cases. This involves surgical fusion of the hip joint ultimately providing symptomatic relief in young patients with advanced arthritis and reduced mobility. However, individuals usually develop spine and knee pain over the years and a conversion of the arthrodesis to a total hip replacement is then indicated.
- In a salvage situation, an excision arthroplasty (Girdlestone's excision arthroplasty) may be indicated. This involves excision of the femoral head.

KEY POINTS

- Osteoarthritis of the hip presents with pain located in the groin/buttock and/or radiating to the knee.
- Clinical signs are an antalgic gait, positive Trendelenburg sign, unequal leg length, muscle wasting, and a restriction of hip joint movements.
- It most commonly affects middle-aged and elderly individuals.
- Imaging should be an anteroposterior standing hip X-ray and a lateral view of the affected hip.
- Management is initially conservative. Surgery includes total joint replacement.

CASE 27: LATERAL HIP PAIN

History

A 53-year-old woman joined a gym to improve her fitness after putting on a fair amount of weight since her fiftieth birthday. After three weeks of working out she developed right lateral hip pain which was not improving. To her general practitioner she complained of pain that was aggravated by lying on the right side. She could remember no trauma, fever or stiffness in her hips. She also denied any pain in her back or knees.

Examination

Assessment of her gait reveals no limp and she has a negative Trendelenburg sign. On palpation of her right greater trochanter she complains of marked tenderness. Examination of her hip reveals a full range of movement. Plain X-rays do not show any signs of arthritis, with good joint space in the hip joint. The MRI scan is shown in Fig. 27.1.

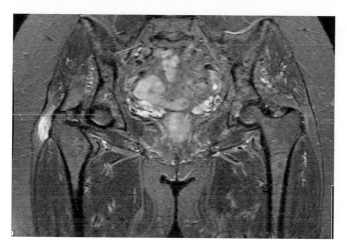

Figure 27.1

Questions

- What is the diagnosis?
- How would you treat this condition?

ANSWER 27

The diagnosis is trochanteric bursitis which typically produces lateral hip pain that is tender to palpation – as in this case. Greater trochanteric pain syndrome (GTPS) is now being commonly substituted for the term trochanteric bursitis.

Trochanteric bursitis refers specifically to inflammation of the trochanteric bursa. The bursa functions normally to minimize friction between the greater trochanter and the iliotibial band, which passes over the bursa with various degrees of hip flexion. Variations in anatomy, such as a broad pelvis, or excessive repetitive contact between the greater trochanter and a tight iliotibial band such as in runners may result in irritation of the bursa and generate pain. Patients typically will have tenderness over the greater trochanter with direct palpation. Pain may radiate down the lateral aspect of the thigh. Generally, if a patient has point tenderness over the greater trochanter, this is suggestive of greater trochanteric bursitis. Bursal swelling may be present, but this may be difficult to appreciate in many patients. Lateral hip pain can be reproduced with flexion of the hip followed by resisted hip abduction. Trochanteric bursitis seems to be much more common in females than in males. MRI and ultrasonographic scans potentially can be employed to differentiate gluteus medius tendinitis from trochanteric bursitis.

Often, trochanteric bursitis is managed non-operatively. First-line management includes relative rest from offending activities, iliotibial band and tensor fascia lata stretching, gluteal muscle strengthening, and anti-inflammatory drugs. Second-line treatment may include modalities such as ultrasound with various degrees of success. If these fail or if a patient cannot tolerate the symptoms, then a local anaesthetic and steroid injection into the point of maximal tenderness is the next step. Radiological confirmation with fluoroscopy or ultrasound improves accuracy of trochanteric bursa injections. Advise the patient to avoid lying on the affected side, if possible.

The majority of patients will improve with conservative management. Surgical intervention should be reserved for individuals who fail to improve from non-operative treatment. Surgery can be undertaken either open or arthroscopically. Surgery involves a release of the iliotibial band in combination with a trochanteric bursectomy.

 KEY POINTS

- In trochanteric bursitis there is tenderness over the greater trochanter with direct palpation.
- It is more common in females than in males.
- Local anaesthetic and steroid injection into the point of maximal tenderness under image guidance is the treatment of choice.

CASE 28: A PAINFUL RED SWOLLEN KNEE

History

A 55-year-old carpet layer has suffered a painful red swelling on the front of his right knee while involved in some intensive contract work (Fig. 28.1). There is no history of trauma. He does not have any fever and appears systemically well. The swelling is not improving and is preventing him from kneeling because of the pain.

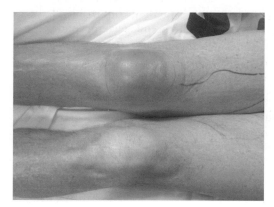

Figure 20.1

Examination

There is some erythema overlying the affected knee. On palpation the knee is warm to the touch and there is a localized lump over the anterior aspect of the patella. The lump is fluctuant in nature and tender to touch. Assessment of the range of movement of the knee reveals a full pain-free range of movement.

Questions
- What is the diagnosis?
- What are the common causes of this condition?
- How would you treat this patient?

ANSWER 28

This man has pre-patellar bursitis (also known as housemaid's knee). It is not septic arthritis as he maintains a full range of movement of his knee joint (in the presence of septic arthritis, with infection and pus in the joint, he would be unable to flex his knee). The pre-patellar bursa is a superficial bursa with a thin synovial lining located between the skin and the patella. The function of the bursa is to reduce friction and allow maximal range of motion.

The causes of pre-patellar bursitis include direct trauma (e.g. following a fall or direct blow to the knee), recurrent overuse such as repeated kneeling, and sepsis secondary to a direct break in the skin. Occupations that are at risk of developing bursitis include carpet layers, priests and housemaids.

Treatment in the acute stage consists of rest. Kneeling should be avoided and protected knee caps advised at work. Non-steroidal anti-inflammatory drugs help to reduce the inflammation. Consider aspiration of the bursa in non-infected cases, particularly if the bursa is large. Incision and drainage of the pre-patellar bursa is usually performed when symptoms of septic bursitis have not improved significantly within 36–48 hours. Surgical removal of the bursa (bursectomy) may be necessary for chronic or recurrent pre-patellar bursitis. In chronic cases, the lump can be excised.

 KEY POINTS

- The function of the pre-patellar bursa is to reduce friction.
- Treatment in the acute stage consists of rest and non-steroidal anti-inflammatory drugs (NSAIDs).

CASE 29: SWELLING IN THE BACK OF THE KNEE

History

A 66-year-old retired man has presented to his general practitioner with a swelling at the back of one of his knees. The lump is not causing him any pain or discomfort, and he is not sure how long it has been there. On further questioning he states that over the last two or three years he has had some early morning stiffness in the knee.

Examination

This man walks with a slight limp. He has a mild varus deformity of the knee and there is an obvious swelling at the back of the knee in the region of the popliteal fossa. The swelling is approximately 3 cm in diameter. The lump is painless to palpation, cool, non-pulsatile, non-tender and fluctuant. It is located in the midline and below the level of the knee joint. There is reduced range of flexion and he is unable to fully extend this knee compared to the other. On palpation, he complains of some tenderness along the medial and lateral joint lines. Assessment of medial and lateral stability reveals a correctable varus deformity and stable ligaments. MRI scans are shown in Figs 29.1 and 29.2.

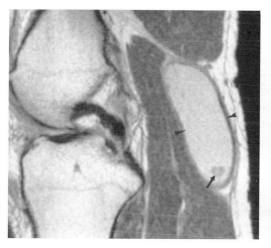

Figure 29.1

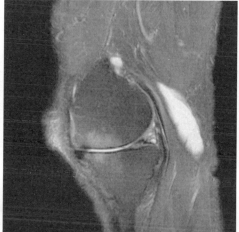

Figure 29.2

Questions

- What is the diagnosis?
- What is the differential diagnosis?
- What is the natural history of these lesions?
- How would you manage this condition?

ANSWER 29

This man has a popliteal (Baker's) cyst. The name of the cyst is in memory of the physician who originally described the condition, the British surgeon William Morrant Baker (1839–96).

The cyst results from fluid distension of the gastrocnemio-semimembranosus bursa. The cyst is located posterior to the medial femoral condyle, between the tendons of the medial head of the gastrocnemius and semimembranosus muscles. It usually communicates with the joint by way of a slit-like opening at the posteromedial aspect of the knee capsule just superior to the joint line. The lesion is typically associated with osteoarthritis in the knee (as in this case), with pain and stiffness. A Baker's cyst is the most common mass in the popliteal fossa.

The differential diagnosis includes lumps arising from the posterior aspect of the knee, with swelling from anatomical structures such as:

- skin and subcutaneous tissue (lipoma, sebaceous cyst)
- artery (popliteal artery aneurysm)
- vein (deep vein thrombosis, saphena varix at saphenopopliteal junction)
- nerve (neuroma)
- enlarged bursae (semimembranosus, medial head of grastrocnemius)
- cyst (Baker's cyst).

In most cases a Baker's cyst is asymptomatic. It is usually associated with rheumatoid arthritis or osteoarthritis. The prevalence of Baker's cysts in patients with inflammatory arthritis is higher than in patients with osteoarthritis. The most common complication of a Baker's cyst is rupture of fluid into the adjacent proximal gastrocnemius muscle, which results in a pseudo-thrombophlebitis syndrome mimicking symptoms of a deep vein thrombosis. The incidence of Baker's cyst rupture is 3–10 per cent.

The diagnosis is confirmed by ultrasound. The scan identifies fluid between the semimembranosus and the medial gastrocnemius tendons. Ultrasonography is useful to determine whether the popliteal mass is a pure cystic structure or a complex cyst and/or solid mass. On MRI, a Baker's cyst appears as a homogeneous, high-signal-intensity, cystic mass behind the medial femoral condyle; a thin, fluid-filled neck interdigitates between the tendons of the medial head of the gastrocnemius and semimembranosus muscles.

Once the diagnosis has been confirmed this can be treated conservatively. The swelling can reduce following aspiration and application of hydrocortisone. Excision is not advised as the rate of recurrence is high. When cartilage tears or other internal knee problems are associated, surgery can be the best treatment option.

 KEY POINTS

- Baker's cyst is fluid distension of the gastrocnemio-semimembranosus bursa.
- Baker's cyst is the most common mass in the popliteal fossa.
- It is associated with arthritis in the knee.
- The diagnosis is confirmed by ultrasound.

CASE 30: A MILDLY SWOLLEN KNEE IN A YOUNG MAN

History

A 25-year-old man was playing football for his local team. While going in for a tackle he sustained a twisting injury to his knee. There was no immediate swelling. He continued to play for about ten minutes to the end of the game but then complained of some pain in the medial aspect of his knee. He awoke the next day with a painful swelling in the knee and so consults his general practitioner.

Examination

This young man has some mild swelling, associated with marked tenderness to palpation over the medial joint line. He has normal varus/valgus stability of the knee and a negative anterior draw and Lachman's test. The range of motion is full. A plain X-ray shows good preservation of the joint space, and an MRI film is shown in Fig. 30.1.

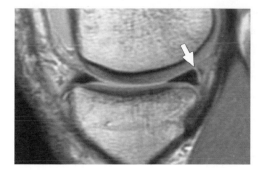

Figure 30.1

Questions

- What is the diagnosis?
- What are the common clinical features of this injury?
- How would you manage this injury?

ANSWER 30

The diagnosis is a tear of the medial meniscus. Meniscus tears typically occur as a result of twisting or change of position of the weight-bearing knee in varying degrees of flexion or extension. The swelling often takes a few hours to become apparent. In contrast, in the presence of an anterior cruciate ligament (ACL) rupture, swelling often occurs immediately or shortly after the injury. This is because the blood vessels in the ACL tend to rupture and cause acute haemarthrosis. Immediate swelling with a meniscal tear indicates a tear in the peripheral vascular aspect, and degenerative tears often manifest with recurrent effusions due to synovitis.

Pain from meniscus injuries is commonly intermittent and is usually the result of synovitis or abnormal motion of the unstable meniscus fragment. The pain is typically localized to the joint line on palpation. In the presence of a large tear the patient can present with a locked knee: the femoral condyle gets trapped within the tear and this prevents the knee from straightening.

Provocative manoeuvres to detect the presence of a tear are based on causing impingement of the torn meniscus between the femoral and tibial surfaces. The McMurray test is positive in the presence of a meniscal tear if you can elicit pain or a reproducible click. The medial meniscus is evaluated by extending the fully flexed knee with the foot and tibia internally rotated while a varus stress is applied. The lateral meniscus is evaluated by extending the knee from the fully flexed position, with the foot/tibia externally rotated while a valgus stress is applied to the knee. One of the examiner's hands should be palpating the joint line during the manoeuvre. Alternatively, Apley's test is performed with the patient prone and the knee flexed 90 degrees. An axial load is applied through the heel as the lower leg is internally and externally rotated. This grinding manoeuvre is suggestive of meniscal pathology if pain is elicited at the medial or lateral joint line.

The natural history of a short (<1 cm) vascular, longitudinal tear is often one of healing or resolution of symptoms. Stable tears with minimal displacement, degenerative tears, or partial-thickness tears may become asymptomatic with non-operative management. Surgical treatment of symptomatic meniscal tears is recommended because untreated tears may increase in size and may abrade articular cartilage, resulting in arthritis. Symptomatic meniscal tears usually respond well to arthroscopic surgical treatment in the absence of arthritis. Partial meniscectomy is the treatment of choice for tears in the avascular portion of the meniscus or complex tears that are not amenable to repair. Torn tissue is removed, and the remaining healthy meniscal tissue is contoured to a stable, balanced peripheral rim.

Types of meniscus tears are:

- longitudinal tears that may take the shape of a bucket handle if displaced
- radial tears
- parrot-beak or oblique flap tears
- horizontal tears
- complex tears that combine variants of the above.

Resection of part of the meniscus can increase contact pressure significantly. Meniscus repair is recommended for tears that occur in the peripheral vascular region (red zone or red–white zone), are longer than 1 cm, involve greater than 50 per cent of the meniscal thickness, and are unstable to arthroscopic probing. The red zone is the well-vascularized periphery, the red–white zone is the middle portion with vascularity peripherally but not centrally, and the white zone is the central avascular portion. A stable knee is important for successful meniscus repair and healing. In the long term, meniscal repairs fail to heal in 5–10 per cent of patients.

 KEY POINTS

- Medial meniscal tears occur with a compression and twisting mechanism.
- Assess tenderness to palpation of the joint line.
- Repair tears in red–red and red–white zones.
- Resect tears in the white–white zone.

CASE 31: AN ATRAUMATIC PAINFUL KNEE IN AN ELDERLY WOMAN

History

A 73-year-old woman presents with left knee pain. This pain has gradually deteriorated over the last three years. She reports early-morning stiffness in the knee. Her walking distance has reduced significantly and is limited due to pain. She obtains minimal relief with analgesia and rest. She has noticed some swelling in the knee and finds walking over uneven surfaces painful, and she finds going down stairs difficult. She has developed pain at night that keeps her awake. She has no history of trauma or infection. She reports no pain in her hips or back.

Examination

This woman has valgus (knock) knees with the left more affected than the right, associated with an effusion. She has an antalgic gait. She has marked tenderness over the lateral joint line and crepitus in the patellofemoral joint. She has flexion from 5 to 85 degrees with correctable valgus deformity. Radiographs are shown in Figs 31.1 and 31.2.

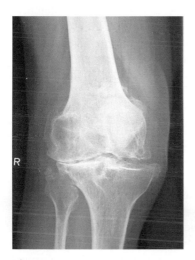

Figure 31.1

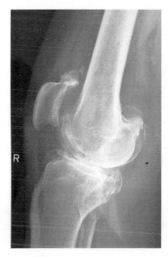

Figure 31.2

Questions

- What is the diagnosis?
- Describe the radiological signs in the right knee joint.
- What are the management options?

ANSWER 31

The diagnosis is osteoarthritis of the knee characterized by the pain, early-morning stiffness, deformity and radiographic findings. This elderly woman has insidious pain in the knee. There was no pre-existing event to explain the pain. Early-morning stiffness that gradually diminishes with activity is typical of osteoarthritis.

The bones forming the knee joint comprise the femur, tibia and patella. The femur and tibia converge towards the knee at approximately 5–7 degrees. Greater angles result in genu valgum which is more common in females, and a lesser angle results in genu varum which is more common in males. The patient has a 5-degree flexion contracture which is commonly caused by posterior osteophytes on the femur, loose body and contracture of the posterior knee capsule. Normal knee flexion is to 130 degrees and flexion to only 85 degrees is not uncommon with arthritis. Tenderness in the joint lines suggests that the menisci are affected. It is important to assess the stability of the knee by testing the medial and collateral ligaments as well as the integrity of the anterior and posterior cruciate ligaments. As part of your examination, pathology in the joints above and below should be excluded. Patients with degenerative hip disease may present with referred pain through the obturator nerve to the medial side of the knee.

The radiological signs include joint space narrowing in the lateral and patellofemoral joint. This is associated with subchondral sclerosis and osteophyte formation (bony outgrowths covered by hyaline cartilage that typically develop at the margins of the joints). Often subchondral cyst formation also occurs. In degenerative arthritis the quality of the articular cartilage is lost. Early in the process, there may be discrete chondral injuries, whereas advanced changes include injuries on both sides of the joint. The cartilage surface becomes thin and sometimes denuded. The subchondral bone becomes thickened, sclerotic and polished (eburnated). Cysts may arise from increased intra-articular synovial fluid pressure.

During the initial stages the management of knee osteoarthritis is conservative. This comprises oral analgesia such as non-steroidal anti-inflammatory drugs. These help to regulate the inflammatory response and can reduce disease symptoms. Steroid, visco supplementation injections and local heat can also be used. Although steroid injections can provide transient relief, they can also lead to cartilage destruction with recurrent injections. A reduction of cartilage impact loading can be reduced by using a walking stick, cushioned heels and weight loss. Knee bracing can be helpful with a correctable deformed knee. Physiotherapy can improve the strength of the extensor mechanism.

When conservative management fails to relieve symptoms then surgery can be considered. Initially, joint-preserving surgery can be considered in the absence of severe arthritis. The options include an arthroscopic debridement. However, in a recent report in *The Lancet*, the outcomes after arthroscopic lavage or debridement were no better than after a placebo procedure. Bone realignment procedures such as high tibial osteotomy are an option in the presence of unicompartmental early degenerative disease. The osteotomy helps redistribute the loads to the uninvolved compartment. Joint replacement options include partial or total. Unicompartmental joint replacement is indicated in patients with single compartment disease. The results are good if the indications for surgery are adhered to. Patellofemoral arthroplasty is sometimes indicated in isolated patellofemoral disease in young patients and is a relatively new procedure. Finally, the most common strategy for joint replacement and most widely adopted is a total knee replacement. Joint replacement surgery should aim to correct deformity, improve the painful symptoms and improve mobility.

KEY POINTS

- Genu valgum is more common in females and genu varum is more common in males.
- Radiological signs of knee osteoarthritis are joint space narrowing, subchondral sclerosis, osteophyte formation and subchondral cyst formation.
- Initial management is conservative with oral analgesia such as NSAIDs.
- Steroid injections can provide transient relief, but they can also lead to cartilage destruction with recurrent injections.
- Physiotherapy can improve strength.

CASE 32: AN UNSTABLE KNEE IN A YOUNG MAN

History

A 22-year-old man was playing football and had to suddenly change direction. He heard a pop in his leg, which suddenly gave way. Immediately after this he noticed a large swelling had developed in the knee and he was unable to finish the game. Six weeks later the main swelling had subsided, but his knee felt unstable and kept giving way when he tried to run or suddenly change direction. He went to his general practitioner.

Examination

This young man's knee is moderately swollen. He has no palpable tenderness in his joint line and medial or lateral instability. However, assessment of his knee in the antero-posterior (AP) plane reveals signs of instability. Plain X-rays of the knee look normal with no evidence of a fracture. An MRI scan is shown in Fig. 32.1.

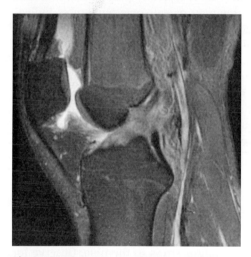

Figure 32.1

Questions

- What is the diagnosis?
- What clinical tests would you do to assess stability of the knee?
- What associated injuries can occur?
- What is the management of this injury?

ANSWER 32

The diagnosis is a ruptured anterior cruciate ligament (ACL) which is a typical injury associated with immediate swelling and instability of the knee. The ACL attaches the femur to the tibia. The ACL has anteromedial and posterolateral bands which are affected by movement. During flexion, the anterior band is taut, and the posterior band is loose. However, during extension, the posterolateral band is tight, while the anterior band is loose. The tibial attachment is wider and stronger than the femoral attachment. The ACL receives nerve fibres from the posterior branch of the posterior tibial nerve. The main function of these nerves is believed to be proprioception. The ACL is the primary restraint to limit anterior translation of the tibia. The greatest restraint is in full extension. The ACL also serves as a secondary restraint to tibial rotation and varus/valgus angulation at full extension. When the ACL is injured, a combination of anterior translation and rotation occurs.

During the initial assessment, look for an effusion. This is typically present and indicates intra-articular pathology. Palpation of the joint line may reveal some tenderness indicative of a meniscal tear. Assessment of the range of movement and noting a lack of full extension may indicate a bucket-handle tear of the meniscus or loose body. Assess the mediolateral stability particularly during valgus stress looking for an injury to the medial collateral ligament. The most sensitive test looking for anterior cruciate ligament laxity is the Lachman test. The knee should be placed in 30 degrees of flexion. With one hand, stabilize the femur and with the other hand direct a force to the back of the calf anteriorly. Observe the amount of displacement and the quality of the end-point. Comparison to the other knee may reveal some asymmetry and greater than 3 mm is considered abnormal.

The least sensitive test is the anterior draw test. This test is performed with the knee flexed to 90 degrees. The examiner should sit gently on the patient's foot and hold the calf with both hands. Apply an anterior force and any anterior tibial excursion should be compared to the other side.

Under a general anaesthetic the pivot shift test is useful. Perform the test with the leg extended and the foot in internal rotation. Apply a valgus stress to the tibia. Observe for a reduction of the anteriorly subluxed tibia at approximately 30 degrees.

Radiological investigations should comprise AP, lateral, skyline and notch views to exclude any bony fractures. MRI has a sensitivity of 90–98 per cent for ACL tears and is also useful for detecting any associated meniscal tears.

Approximately 50 per cent of patients with ACL injuries also have meniscal tears. In acute ACL injuries, the lateral meniscus is more commonly torn; in chronic ACL tears, the medial meniscus is more commonly torn. The ACL-deficient knee has also been linked to an increased rate of degenerative changes and meniscal injuries.

The classic 'terrible triad' (anterior and medial cruciate ligaments, plus medial meniscus tears) involves a valgus stress to the knee with resultant acute injury to the ACL and MCL. However, the medial meniscus tear is now thought to occur later, as a result of chronic ACL deficiency.

Conservative management is typically reserved for individuals who do not participate in sports or are not involved in heavy manual work. Reconstruction is often considered following a trial of conservative management in patients with instability.

KEY POINTS

- The ACL is the primary restraint to limit anterior translation of the tibia.
- The most sensitive test looking for anterior cruciate ligament laxity is the Lachman test.
- MRI has a sensitivity of 90–98 per cent for ACL tears.
- Treatment options include conservative, physiotherapy and finally reconstruction.

CASE 33: AN INJURED ANKLE

History

A 39-year-old businessman recently took up squash in his leisure time. He started to complain of mild pain in the posterior aspect of his ankle while playing. Then, while playing, he heard a sudden snap in the lower calf associated with severe pain. He was able to walk with a limp, but unable to run or stand on his toes and had to stop playing immediately. He is otherwise fit and well and his only recent medication has been a course of a fluoroquinolone for a chest infection.

Examination

This man's affected ankle has some swelling over the posterior aspect. On palpation, he has some tenderness over the Achilles tendon and a palpable gap. With the patient prone, squeezing the calf demonstrates no passive plantar flexion of the foot.

Questions
- What is the diagnosis?
- What are the risk factors?
- What clinical and radiological tests are useful to confirm the diagnosis?
- What are the options for treatment?

ANSWER 33

The diagnosis is a ruptured Achilles tendon, characterized by a history of a sudden snap and no passive plantarflexion of the foot while the calf is squeezed.

The Achilles tendon is the largest and strongest tendon in the human body, and it is formed from tendinous contributions of the gastrocnemius and soleus muscles. The tendons converge approximately 15 cm proximal to the insertion at the posterior calcaneus. The tendon has the ability to stretch by up to 4 per cent before damage occurs. With stretch greater than 8 per cent, macroscopic rupture occurs. The blood supply for the tendon is derived from the posterior tibial artery. The watershed zone is an area 2–6 cm proximal to the calcaneus, in which the blood supply is less abundant and becomes even sparser with age. It is in this region that most degeneration and therefore rupture of the tendon occurs. The differential diagnosis is soft-tissue or bony pathology. Soft-tissue pathology includes Achilles peritendonitis (tends to have some activity-related pain, swelling and sometimes crepitus along the tendon sheath with nodularity), tendinosis (characterized by mucoid degeneration of the tendon with a lack of inflammatory response), or gastrocnemius or soleus tear. Bony pathology includes calcaneal bony injury or inflammatory arthropathy.

There is a risk in men between the ages of 30 and 50 years who are generally recreational athletes. An activity involving a sudden forceful contraction of the Achilles tendon can cause a rupture. Other mechanisms include direct trauma. Up to 50 per cent of ruptures have had a history of pre-existing chronic tendonitis. Corticosteroid injection of the Achilles tendon or its sheath has been implicated as the cause of subsequent tendon rupture. Another risk factor is the use of fluoroquinolone antibiotics.

The majority of Achilles tendon tears occur in the left leg in the substance of the tendo Achilles, approximately 2–6 cm (the 'watershed zone') above the calcaneal insertion of the tendon. This zone is relatively hypovascular. Clinical examination of the tendon may reveal tenderness, swelling (at the rupture site or more proximally in the calf), bruising, and a palpable gap in the Achilles tendon. There is a loss of plantar flexion power in the foot and the patient will not be able to stand on tip-toes.

A special test for Achilles tendon rupture is the Thompson test. The patient is positioned prone; squeezing the calf of the extended leg may demonstrate no passive plantar flexion of the foot if its Achilles tendon is ruptured. Investigations that are useful to diagnose the rupture include ultrasound or MRI. Ultrasound can assess the tendon thickness and the presence of a tear. Imaging the tendon tear in the plantarflexed position also allows assessment of whether the two ends are apposed or whether there is a gap. MRI is useful in incomplete rupture and is helpful in the assessment of paratendonitis and tendinosis. Plain radiogrphs are useful if you suspect a calcaneal fracture.

Treatment options, non-operative or operative, are determined on a patient-by-patient basis. The average time for immobilization in a cast is about 9 weeks.

KEY POINTS

- The watershed vascular zone of the Achilles tendon is an area 2–6 cm proximal to the calcaneus.
- The Thompson test is useful for Achilles tendon rupture.
- Ultrasound scanning is the initial investigation of choice.
- Treat using a plaster cast when the tendon edges are apposed, and surgery when there is a gap.

CASE 34: DEFORMED FEET IN A NEWBORN CHILD

History

A 30-year-old woman at 40 weeks' gestation delivers a baby after a 16-hour period of labour. The parents think that both the baby's feet look abnormal. The paediatrician is called to assess the newborn's feet.

Examination

The positions of both feet are in equinus and the feet are also supinated and adducted (Fig. 34.1). The feet are not tender, and the overlying skin looks healthy. Pulses are present.

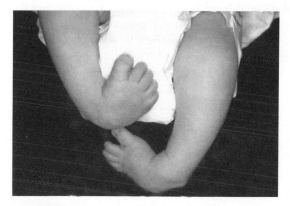

Figure 34.1

Questions

- What is the diagnosis?
- Describe the deformity.
- What are the principles of conservative treatment?

ANSWER 34

The diagnosis is club feet (congenital talipes equinovarus, CTEV), which is a structural deformity present at birth. The deformity is maintained by a combination of contracted joint capsule ligaments and contracted foot and ankle ligaments. Club foot can be classified as either postural or fixed. Fixed or rigid club feet are either flexible (correctable without surgery) or resistant (correctable with surgery). Club foot is bilateral in about 50 per cent of cases and occurs in approximately 1 in 800 births. The condition is more common in males with a 2:1 ratio, and there is a 10 per cent chance of a subsequent baby being affected if the parents already have one child affected.

The bones of the midfoot are affected. The navicular is displaced medially, as is the cuboid. Contractures of the medial plantar soft tissues are present. The talar neck is easily palpable in the sinus tarsi as it is uncovered laterally. Normally, this is covered by the navicular, and the talar body is in the mortise. The medial malleolus is difficult to palpate and is often in contact with the navicular. The hindfoot is supinated, but the foot is often in a position of pronation relative to the hindfoot. The first ray often drops to create a position of cavus. The calcaneus also sits in equinus with the anterior aspect rotated medially and the posterior aspect laterally. The heel is small and feels empty and soft to touch. As the treatment progresses, the calcaneal position improves and the heel begins to feel firm.

The goal of treatment is to obtain a functional plantigrade cosmetically acceptable painless foot. In the present case, non-operative treatment comprised the Ponseti method which is used to correct the cavus, the adduction, then varus, and lastly the equinus deformity (CAVE). Splintage begins at 2–3 days after birth. The foot should be re-manipulated weekly and reassessed radiographically at 3 months. An Achilles tenotomy may be necessary if the hindfoot equinus persists. Surgery should be used as soon as it is obvious that conservative treatment is failing. Operative treatments involve soft-tissue release for children (6–12 months). These include posterior release or complete soft-tissue releases such as posteromedial plantar release or complete subtalar release. Other procedures used include tendon transfers, tibialis anterior, and bone procedures, osteotomies and arthrodeses. Orthoses, Denis Browne bars and Bebax shoes are used to maintain the correction.

 KEY POINTS

- Club foot is a structural deformity present at birth.
- Feet can be assessed and scored using the Pirani scoring system.
- Club feet are either flexible (correctable without surgery) or resistant (correctable with surgery).
- The goal of treatment is to obtain a functional, plantigrade, cosmetically acceptable and painless foot.
- Non-operative treatment comprises the Ponseti method. Operative treatments comprise soft-tissue release, osteotomies and tendon transfers.

CASE 35: HIGH-ARCHED FEET IN A YOUNG GIRL

History

A 9-year-old girl and her grandmother went shopping for new shoes. The girl was having trouble getting her toes into the conventional shoes because they were rubbing on top of the shoes. Her grandmother noticed that the shape of her granddaughter's feet was similar in appearance to her husband's, and there was a family history of Charcot–Marie–Tooth (CMT) disease. The following day they go to see their general practitioner.

Examination

Both feet have high medial arches and there appears to be bilateral clawing of the fore-foot toes. On palpation, she had tenderness under the metatarsal heads with some callosities (Fig. 35.1).

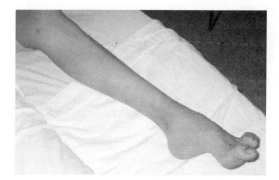

Figure 35.1

Questions
- Describe the deformity in the feet.
- What are the causes of this condition?
- How would you examine this patient's feet?

ANSWER 35

The girl has a cavus deformity of the feet (pes cavus) with an elevated longitudinal arch due to fixed plantarflexion of the forefoot. Associated deformities include claw toes. The deformity can be located in the forefoot, midfoot, hindfoot, or a combination thereof. The main type of cavus foot is the cavovarus deformity. In CMT, the anterior tibialis muscle and the peroneus muscle develop weaknesses. Antagonist muscles, posterior tibialis and peroneus longus, pull harder than the other muscles, causing deformity. Specifically, the peroneus longus pulls harder than the weak anterior tibialis, causing plantarflexion of the first ray and forefoot valgus. The posterior tibialis pulls harder than the weak peroneus brevis, causing forefoot adduction. Intrinsic muscle develops contractures while the long extensor to the toes, recruited to assist in ankle dorsiflexion, causes cock-up or claw-toe deformity – as in this case. With the forefoot valgus and the hindfoot varus, increased stress is placed on the lateral ankle ligaments and instability can occur.

With a unilateral deformity, possible causes are cerebral palsy, diastematoyelia, spinal cord tumour or tethered cord. With a bilateral deformity, possible causes are neuromuscular diseases such as Becker's muscular dystrophy, cerebral palsy, congenital pes cavus, CMT, dystonia, Friedreich's ataxia or poliomyelitis.

The deformity is assessed to discover whether it is flexible or rigid. The forefoot is observed for plantar flexion, and the hindfoot is observed for varus. A full neurological examination documenting the strength of the individual muscles is essential for determining surgical options. Assess the hindfoot flexibility of a cavovarus foot using the Coleman block test. This test is useful to assess hindfoot flexibility and pronation of the forefoot. The test is performed by placing the patient's foot on the block and asking them to bear full weight. The first, second and third metatarsals should be allowed to hang freely into plantarflexion and pronation. This effectively negates the effect of the first metatarsal in plantarflexion on the hindfoot. If the hindfoot varus corrects, while standing on the block, the hindfoot is considered flexible.

If the subtalar joint is flexible and corrects with the Coleman block test, then surgery can be directed to the forefoot. However, if the subtalar joint is rigid, then surgical correction of both the forefoot and hindfoot should be considered.

 KEY POINTS

- Pes cavus is an elevated longitudinal arch due to fixed plantarflexion of the forefoot.
- The forefoot is observed for plantarflexion, and the hindfoot is observed for varus.
- A full neurological examination documenting the strength of the individual muscles should be performed, plus the Coleman block test.
- Orthotics with extra-depth shoes to off-load bony prominences and prevent rubbing of the toes may improve symptoms.

CASE 36: FLAT FEET IN A YOUNG GIRL

History

A mother suspected that her 5-year-old daughter's feet were both too flat. The girl was not, however, complaining of any pain and was walking and running normally. Nevertheless the mother takes her to see the general practitioner because her son's feet are not flat. The girl is fit and healthy.

Examination

This child walks without a limp and has flattening of the medial arches (Figs 36.1 and 36.2). When she is asked to stand on tip-toes there is restoration of the medial arches in both feet. A radiograph is shown in Fig. 36.3.

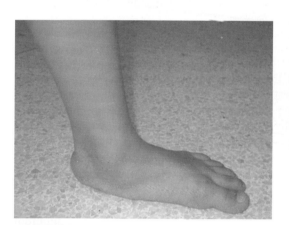

Figure 36.1

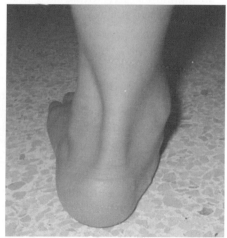

Figure 36.2

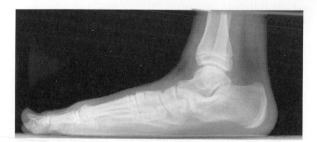

Figure 36.3

Questions

- Describe the deformity in the feet.
- Describe the stages of this condition.
- What investigations would you offer, and why?
- What are the causes of this condition?

ANSWER 36

The diagnosis is flat feet deformity (pes planus). The clinical presentation can be extremely variable and directly correlates with the stage of the disease.

The deformity involves 'shortening' of the lateral column, plantar inclination of the talar head, and lateral subluxation of the navicular on the talar head. Clinically, the arch flattens, the forefoot abducts (the 'too-many-toes' sign), and heel valgus occurs – as in this case. Clinical manifestations that ensue include the inability to perform a single-leg heel rise. This inability to invert the heel results in chronic heel valgus and subsequent Achilles contracture.

Typically infants have a minimal arch and often toddlers have flattening of the long arch, forefoot pronation and heel valgus. Usually these children spontaneously develop a strong normal arch within their first decade. The majority of feet improve as the child ages, at least until 5–6 years old.

There are three stages.

- In stage 1, mild tenderness occurs along the inframalleolar course of the posterior tibial tendon (PTT), with minimal (if any) loss in tendon strength as assessed by the single-limb, heel-rise test. When the patient bears weight only on the involved extremity, performing the heel-rise test demonstrates not only adequate strength but also initiation of heel inversion, which signals an intact tendon.
- Stage 2 disease is a dynamic deformity, where there is hindfoot valgus with forefoot abduction. Palpation along the course of the PTT demonstrates pain. Observing the patient's stance from behind reveals increased visualization of the lateral toes (too-many-toes sign) on the affected extremity secondary to weakness. Single-limb heel rise may not be possible due to weakness, and if performed, corrective heel inversion is generally absent.
- In stage 3, chronic dysfunction and lengthening of the PTT lead to fixed hindfoot deformity. In order to achieve a plantigrade foot in the setting of a fixed hindfoot valgus, the forefoot typically compensates into a fixed supination position. With stage 3 disease, patients often present with lateral pain secondary to subfibular impingement as the calcaneus subluxes and the flat-foot deformity progresses.

Recently, a fourth stage has been added to the original description of PTT dysfunction. Longstanding hindfoot valgus places increasing stress on the deltoid complex, with eventual loss of competence. The resultant valgus tilt of the talus leads to eccentric loading of the ankle with subsequent tibiotalar arthrosis.

Three weight-bearing views of the foot are desirable (anteroposterior, oblique, lateral) plus three weight-bearing views of the ankle (AP, mortise, lateral). Evaluation of longitudinal arch collapse is largely dependent on weight-bearing lateral radiographs. The axis of the talar/first metatarsal angle on the lateral weight-bearing foot radiograph is the most discriminating parameter. Alternatively, the distance between the medial cuneiform and the floor is a strong reflection of medial arch collapse and flat foot. Additional features of pes planus deformity that are noted on the lateral view include talar plantar-flexion and decreased calcaneal pitch.

An AP standing foot projection is primarily used for evaluating talar head uncoverage secondary to lateral deviation of the navicular. Also look for evidence of valgus talar tilt with resultant subluxation, arthrosis, or both. The ankle view is particularly important in patients who have fixed hindfoot valgus. MRI provides highly detailed evaluations of the posterior tibial tendon.

Pes planus can be classified as either flexible or rigid. The most common cause is posterior tibial tendon insufficiency. The condition is most common in middle-aged women with obesity. Younger patients who present with rigid pes planus should be screened for conditions such as tarsal coalition and congenital vertical talus.

Patients with asymptomatic pes planus may progress to a symptomatic stage as the degenerative process progresses. Trauma to both the bony and soft tissue of the midfoot can lead to the deformity. Fracture dislocation to the medial column (navicular and first metatarsal) and rupture to the spring ligament or plantar fascia lead to progressive collapse of the medial longitudinal arch. Neuropathy secondary to diabetes mellitus, spinal cord injury and Charcot neuropathy are conditions seen with pes planus.

 KEY POINTS

- Pes planus is divided into rigid and flexible types, and three stages of disease are defined.
- Posterior tibial tendon insufficiency is the most common cause.
- Conservative treatment includes accommodating footwear and insoles. Surgery involves soft-tissue and/or bone procedures.

CASE 37: A PAINFUL AND SWOLLEN ANKLE

History
A 28-year-old man slipped while crossing a road and sustained a pronation–eversion injury to his left ankle. He complained of severe pain immediately in his ankle and hobbled over to the other side of the road.

Examination
This man's ankle is swollen on the medial, anterior and lateral sides. There is some obvious bruising both medially and laterally. Palpation of the medial and lateral aspect of the ankle is very tender. Assessment of movement reveals pain on ankle dorsiflexion and plantarflexion with extreme apprehension and reluctance. He is unable to fully weight-bear on the left ankle owing to pain. A radiograph of the ankle is shown in Fig. 37.1.

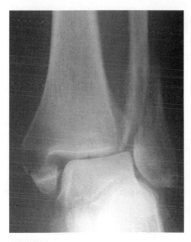

Figure 37.1

Questions
- What is the diagnosis?
- Describe the key ligaments responsible for stability in the ankle.
- What are the principles of management?

ANSWER 37

The diagnosis is a fracture of the fibula and medial malleolus shown by the pain in the lateral and medial malleolus, inability to bear weight, and fracture lines through the fibula and medial malleolus. The fibula fracture is above the level of the ankle syndesmosis. This is an unstable fracture. The Danis–Weber classification is based on the level of the fibular fracture, the level of the tibiofibular syndesmotic disruption and potential talar (ankle) instability (see the box). The initial X-ray includes at least three projections: anteroposterior, lateral and mortise views, with the foot in internal rotation of 15 degrees. Occasionally stress radiographs for lateral or medial instability may be necessary. Greater than 5 mm of medial clear joint space seen on static or stress radiographs indicates injury to the deltoid ligament.

The ankle is a modified hinge joint with three bones (tibia, fibula and talus) and the ligaments that bind these bones as a unit. The lateral collateral ligament consists of three components: anterior talofibular ligament (ATFL), calcaneofibular ligament (CFL), and posterior talofibular ligament (PTFL). On the medial side, the deltoid ligament consists of a superficial and a deep stronger portion and is in the main a medial stabilizer of the ankle joint. The distal end of the fibula lies against the tibial groove, held together by a complex of distal tibiofibular ligaments and is called a syndesmosis. This complex consists of a group of ligaments: anteroinferior and posteroinferior tibiofibular ligaments and the strongest one, the interosseous ligament, which is the thickest part of the interosseous membrane.

Closed reduction with below-knee cast immobilization should be reserved for undisplaced, stable fractures, anatomically reduced fractures, and for patients with poor medical condition such as elderly diabetics. Unstable fractures or fractures with displacement should be considered for surgical management. The timing of surgery is important. It should either be early, before the ankle swells, or (as in the present case) delayed for 7–10 days to allow the swelling to subside. Most isolated undisplaced Danis–Weber type A fractures can be treated conservatively in a below-knee walking plaster for 6–8 weeks, allowing weight-bearing as tolerated until the fibular has healed. Stable, undisplaced fractures of the malleoli with posterior malleolus involvement of less than 25 per cent of the articular surface can also be treated conservatively with plaster for 6 weeks and non-weight-bearing. Bimalleolar and trimalleolar injuries are unstable and are treated with open reduction and internal fixation. Most displaced medial malleolar fractures should be opened, and the trapped periosteum removed and fixed to restore normal ankle congruency and deltoid integrity.

! | **Danis–Weber classification of fibular fractures**

- Type A: Fibular fracture below the joint line, with intact syndesmosis
- Type B: Fracture at the level of the ankle joint line, with partial syndesmotic injury
- Type C: Fibular fracture proximal to the tibiofibular joint with associated disruption of the syndesmosis. Two subtypes are recognized: diaphyseal (Dupuytren) and proximal (Maisonnevue)

KEY POINTS

- Fibular fractures are classified as Danis–Weber A, B or C.
- Greater than 5 mm of medial clear joint space indicates injury to the deltoid ligament.
- Closed reduction with below-knee cast immobilization should be reserved for undisplaced, stable fractures. Open reduction and internal fixation is used for displaced unstable fractures.

CASE 38: DEFORMED FEET IN AN ELDERLY WOMAN

History

A 70-year-old woman has been having trouble finding comfortable shoes because the shape of her feet has changed over the past few years. She recalls that her mother's feet were similar in shape. She went to see her general practitioner in order to be referred to a foot specialist. She reports an aching pain in her first metatarsophalangeal joint of the right foot while walking. She recalls no history of trauma.

Examination

There is swelling and deformity of the first metatarsophalangeal (MTP) joint with lateral deviation of the great toe. This is associated with overriding of the second toe towards the great toe (Fig. 38.1). A radiograph is shown in Fig. 38.2.

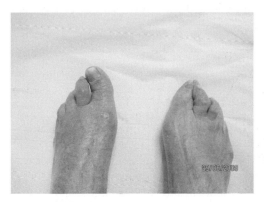

Figure 38.1   Figure 38.2

Questions

- What is the diagnosis?
- Describe the features on physical examination associated with this condition in addition to the lateral deviation of the great toe and overriding second toe.
- What are the options for treatment?

ANSWER 38

The diagnosis is hallux valgus because of the swelling, deformity and associated lateral deviation of the toe. It may be associated with medial deviation of the first ray known as metatarsus primus varus. Pronation of the hallux may also be present.

The physical findings include a bunion which may be inflamed and tender – as in this case. The bunion is typically located over the dorsomedial aspect of the first metatarsal joint. There may be evidence of crepitus in the first MTP joint and some stiffness indicating degenerative changes in the joint. Assess the first metatarsal (MT) cuneiform joint for hypermobility and tenderness by pushing the MT head into dorsiflexion and plantar-flexion. There may be splaying of the forefoot and tenderness to palpation under the lesser metartarsal head (metatarsalgia). Patients will often describe a feeling like walking on pebbles. The lesser toe deformities are associated with hammer toes. The distal inter-phalangeal joints are often associated with corns or callosities on the dorsum of the toes.

Management of hallux valgus is initially non-operative treatment using footwear that accommodates the deformity. Shoes may be modified to provide more width and depth for the forefoot. In the presence of degenerative disease of the MTP joint, a stiff-soled shoe may be beneficial. Padding and strapping have limited benefit in the long term but may be useful in the elderly who are not medically fit for surgery.

If there remains some flexibility in the foot, orthotics may have a role. However, in the presence of rigid deformity the foot cannot be manipulated and will need to be accommodated by the orthosis.

When conservative management fails, surgery is considered. The goals of surgical treatment are to relieve symptoms, restore function, and correct the deformity and prevent recurrence.

 KEY POINTS

- In hallux valgus there is lateral deviation of the great toe and a bunion over the dorsomedial aspect of the first metatarsal joint.
- Assess for crepitus/stiffness in the first MTP joint, metatarsalgia, hammer toes, corns or callosities on the dorsum of the toes.
- Initial management is non-operative treatment using footwear that accommodates the deformity. Surgical management includes a combination of soft-tissue procedures and osteotomies.

CASE 39: A STIFF GREAT TOE

History

A 45-year-old woman has been experiencing a painful right great toe for 4 years. There is no recall of trauma or infection, or history of gout in the great toe, but it is swollen and stiff. The pain is localized to the first metatarsophalangeal (MTP) joint, and is aggravated by activity. The woman is otherwise medically fit and well.

Examination

The first MTP joint shows no signs of erythema. There is a firm dorsal swelling over the MTP joint that is tender to palpation. There is no active or passive dorsiflexion in the first MTP joint. There are no signs of neurovascular deficit. Radiographs of the affected toe are shown in Figs 39.1 and 39.2.

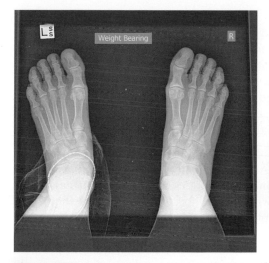

Figure 39.1

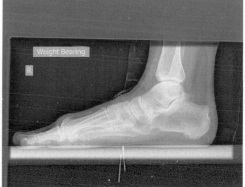

Figure 39.2

Questions
- What is the diagnosis?
- What are the radiological features?
- What are the management options?

ANSWER 39

The diagnosis is hallux rigidus because of the stiffness and presence of dorsal osteophytes seen on the radiographs. This condition encompasses mild to severe degenerative arthritis of the first MTP joint of the foot. The patient complains of pain from impingement of the dorsal osteophytes, especially during walking on rough ground and slopes. The patient may also complain of diffuse, lateral forefoot pain resulting from increased weight-bearing on the lateral foot to offload the hallux. Dorsiflexion is restricted, but the foot may demonstrate compensatory hyperextension of the interphalangeal joint.

Hallux rigidus is the second most common condition affecting the great toe, the first being hallux valgus. The condition is more common in females than males. This condition is seen in two distinct populations: those who present in adolescence and those who present in adulthood. In the adolescent type, localized chondral lesions in the articular surface of the metatarsal head are present. In the adult type, there is more generalized arthritis.

Radiological features include squaring off of the first MTP joint and loss of joint space, osteophytes as seen in the radiographs, cyst formation and sclerosis. The articular degenerative changes are associated with dehydration of the cartilage, which in turn is more susceptible to injury resulting from shear and compressive forces. The subchondral bone shares these stresses, which subsequently lead to increased subchondral bone density, formation of periarticular osteophytes and, in severe cases, cystic changes. The osteophytes limit first MTP joint motion. In severe cases, the articular cartilage is completely denuded.

Initially the management is conservative. Medication options include analgesic and non-steroidal anti-inflammatory drugs (NSAIDs). Mechanical methods limiting the first MTP joint motion are helpful. The use of in-shoe orthotics with medial stiffness, stiff-soled shoes with a rocker bottom, shoes with a wide toe box, low-heeled shoes, and shoe modifications, such as a steel shank placed along the entire medial side, may be beneficial. Activity modifications include avoiding extremes of dorsiflexion of the great toe, such as those caused by kneeling or squatting with the toes in an extended position. Manipulation combined with steroid injection into the joint can be useful in the early stages of the disease.

Conservative management can often be used to successfully treat patients with varying degrees of severity of hallux rigidus. However, in refractory cases the choice of operation depends on the degree of involvement, limitations of the range of movement, and the person's activity level. Surgical options comprising joint-sparing procedures that remove the dorsal osteophyte (chielectomy) are indicated in early disease. Other surgical procedures are bone-cutting (proximal phalanx and/or metatarsal osteotomy) and joint replacement, which can improve joint movement and relieve pain but is not without complications. Joint fusion (arthrodesis), particularly in advanced cases, provides reliable results in individuals involved in strenuous activities.

 KEY POINTS

- Hallux rigidus is associated with mild to severe degenerative arthritis of the first MTP joint of the foot.
- Pain comes from impingement of the dorsal osteophytes.
- Hallux rigidus may present in adolescence or in adulthood.

CASE 40: MISSHAPEN TOE IN A MIDDLE-AGED WOMAN (1)

History

A 40-year-old woman was shopping for shoes for a special occasion. After several hours and several attempts at selecting shoes, she had not found any that would fit comfortably. She attributed this to her third toe. The tip of the toe had changed in appearance lately and was associated with pain because her toe was rubbing against her shoes. She has decided to seek the advice of a foot specialist.

Examination

This woman has a flexion deformity to the third toe at the level of the distal interphalangeal (DIP) joint (Fig. 40.1). There is a callosity on the dorsum of the DIP joint. She has no neurovascular deficit.

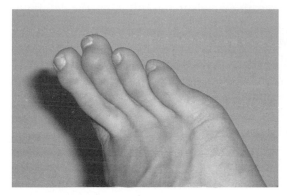

Figure 40.1

Questions

- What is the diagnosis?
- What are the stabilizing factors in the lesser toes?
- How would you manage this patient?

ANSWER 40

This woman has mallet toe deformity which is defined by the flexion deformity of the DIP joint. Mallet toes are common in diabetics with peripheral neuropathy. A mallet deformity is either a flexible or fixed deformity of the distal interphalangeal joint leading to pressure on the tip of the toe, often associated with attenuation of the extensor tendon.

Pain and/or a callosity is often the presenting complaint. This may also lead to nail deformity on the toe. Most commonly the deformity is present in the second toe. A small number of patients can have associated lateral or medial deviation of the toe.

On examination, assess the metatarsophalangeal (MTP) joint, the proximal interphalangeal (PIP) joint, and the location of callosities and nail deformity. Assess the flexibility of the DIP joint with the toe plantarflexed and dorsiflexed at the MTP joint and PIP joint.

The distal interphalangeal joint is a hinge joint with collateral and accessory collateral ligaments and a plantar plate. The flexor sheath extends to the DIP joint. The deformity may be flexible in cases in which the principal problem is an overtight flexor digitorum longus. With fixed deformities the plantar joint structures may be contracted, or alteration of the joint surfaces may have occurred to restrict the joint's range of motion.

Footwear modification such as a wide toe box should be tried first in order to relieve pressure under the tip. Soft orthoses or toe protectors can be useful. Surgical management of mallet toe is indicated if the deformity becomes painful. Surgery comprises a flexor tenotomy, possibly including plantar capsular release and pinning; condylectomy and fusion of the middle to distal phalanx; and, occasionally, partial or complete amputation of the distal phalanx. A flexible mallet toe can be treated with a flexor tenotomy. A fixed deformity can be treated with a condylectomy. An ulcerated or infected toe would do best with a terminal Syme amputation.

 KEY POINTS

- Mallet toe is either a flexible or a fixed deformity of the DIP joint.
- Look for callosities and nail deformity, and assess the flexibility of the DIP joint.
- Footwear modification (e.g. a wide toe box) can be tried initially.
- Surgery comprises a combination of soft-tissue and bony surgery.

CASE 41: MISSHAPEN TOE IN A MIDDLE-AGED WOMAN (2)

History
A 55-year-old woman presents with hardened skin on the dorsal aspect of her second toe. She complains also of occasional pain over the plantar area of the metatarsal head.

Examination
The second toe is flexed at the proximal interphalangeal (PIP) joint. The distal interphalangeal (DIP) joint and metatarsophalangeal (MTP) joint are hyperextended (Fig. 41.1).

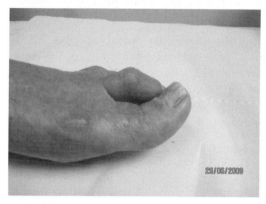

Figure 41.1

Questions
- What is the diagnosis?
- How would you further examine this deformity?
- How would you manage this patient?

ANSWER 41

The diagnosis is hammer toe. Hammer toe deformity is the most common deformity of the lesser toes. The toe is flexed at the PIP joint. The DIP joint and MTP joint are usually hyperextended. The condition often presents with a corn or callosity on the dorsum or the metatarsal head and commonly affects the second toe – as in this case. With progressive PIP joint flexion deformity, compensatory hyperextension of the MTP and DIP joints can occur – as seen in this case. The hyperextension of the MTP joint and flexion of the PIP joint make the PIP joint prominent dorsally. This prominence rubs against the patient's footwear, leading to pain. The deformity is flexible and passively correctable early but typically becomes fixed over time. Progressive deformity can lead to MTP joint dislocation and can be seen on X-rays.

On examination the patient typically complains of pain over the dorsal aspect of the PIP joint. Occasionally, the patient also complains of pain over the plantar area of the metatarsal head, especially if the MTP joint is hyperextended, subluxed or dislocated. A callus may be present over the dorsal surface of the PIP joint, over the plantar surface of the metatarsal head, or at the tip of the toe – as in this case. The extensor digitorum longus (EDL) tendon gradually loses mechanical advantage at the PIP joint, as does the flexor digitorum longus (FDL) tendon at the MTP joint. The intrinsic muscles sublux dorsally as the MTP hyperextends. They now extend the MTP joint and flex the PIP joint, as opposed to their usual functions of flexing the MTP joint and extending the PIP joint.

Examination of hammer toe deformity should include a neurovascular evaluation, including palpation of pulses, a sensory examination, and an evaluation of intrinsic muscle bulk. The deformity should be assessed while the patient is standing. Passive correction of the deformity should be attempted, because this will help determine which treatment options are appropriate for the patient. Diagnostic assessment for hammer toe deformity comprises weight-bearing anteroposterior and lateral radiography of the involved foot. Any intra-articular or periarticular erosions suggest rheumatoid arthritis or psoriatic arthritis, respectively.

The indication for surgical treatment is intractable pain that does not improve with adequate non-operative treatment, including taping (for flexible deformity) and the use of accommodative footwear featuring a toe box of adequate depth (for fixed deformity).

When considering surgery, distinguish between flexible and fixed deformity. If the hammer toe is due to contracture of the FDL tendon, then plantarflexion of the ankle will straighten the toe. In contrast, dorsiflexion of the ankle will worsen the deformity. Flexible deformity of greater magnitude requires a flexor tenotomy. Passively correctable deformity is amenable to tendon transfer procedures such as a Girdlestone–Taylor flexor-to-extensor tendon transfer. A fixed deformity requires at least resection arthroplasty of the PIP joint. The goal is to shorten the toe to decrease the deforming forces of the contracted soft tissues. As the magnitude of the deformity increases, additional procedures may be necessary, such as flexor tenotomy, extensor tenotomy, MTP joint release or arthroplasty, or metatarsal shortening. Both flexible and fixed deformities also may require MTP arthroplasty and/or extensor tenotomy to achieve adequate correction. A metatarsal shortening osteotomy may need to be added for a dislocated MTP joint or MTP instability with synovitis. Plantar condylectomy of the metatarsal head may need to be added for plantar metatarsal head pain without instability or synovitis.

KEY POINTS

- Hammer toe is the most common deformity of the lesser toes.
- The toe is flexed at the PIP joint. The DIP joint and MTP joints are usually hyperextended.
- Non-operative methods are the first line of treatment: taping (for flexible deformity) and the use of accommodative footwear featuring a toe box of adequate depth (for fixed deformity).
- An indication for surgical treatment is intractable pain that does not improve with non-operative treatment.

CASE 42: FOOT PAIN FOLLOWING A RIDING FALL

History
A 45-year-old woman was horse riding when she fell off her mount. As she fell her foot was caught in the stirrup. She complained of an isolated injury with pain in her foot only.

Examination
This woman's left foot has swelling in the midfoot region associated with ecchymosis on the plantar aspect. Palpation of the midfoot is tender, particularly between the first and second metatarsal bases. She has no neurovascular deficit but is unable to bear weight on the foot owing to pain. A radiograph is shown in Fig. 42.1.

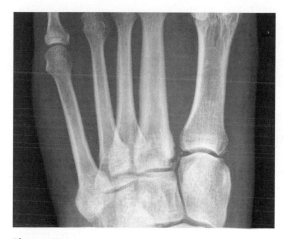

Figure 42.1

Questions
• What is the diagnosis?
• Describe the radiological findings.
• How would you manage this condition?

ANSWER 42

The diagnosis is a Lisfranc injury which is typical with this mechanism of injury. Jacques Lisfranc de Saint-Martin (1790–1847), a field surgeon in Napoleon's army, described an amputation technique across the five tarsometatarsal (TMT) joints. At the time this was an effective solution to forefoot gangrene secondary to frostbite. This anatomical landmark became known as the Lisfranc joint.

The Lisfranc joint, which represents the articulation between the midfoot and forefoot, is composed of the five TMT joints. The Lisfranc ligament is attached to the lateral margin of the medial cuneiform and medial and plantar surface of the second metatarsal (MT) base. This is the only ligamentous support between first and second rays at midfoot level. A Lisfranc injury encompasses everything from a sprain to a complete disruption of normal anatomy through the TMT joints. Injury to this ligament, even in isolation, will result in functional instability with loss of longitudinal and transverse arches. No intermetatarsal ligaments exist between the first and second MTs. Lisfranc injuries are commonly undiagnosed and carry a high risk of chronic secondary disability.

Initial radiographs should include anteroposterior, lateral and oblique views. Standing radiographs are ideal but often too painful. Good alternatives are stress radiographs with the forefoot in dorsiflexion and abduction.

On the radiographs, dislocation of the TMT joint is indicated by loss of in-line arrangement of the lateral margin of the first metatarsal base with the lateral edge of the medial cuneiform; loss of in-line arrangement of the medial margin of the second metatarsal base with the medial edge of the middle cuneiform in the weight-bearing AP view; and the presence of small avulsed fragments ('fleck sign'), which are additional indications of ligamentous injury and probable joint disruption. A fleck sign seen on the AP radiograph is pathognomonic for a Lisfranc injury (present in 90 per cent of instances). It represents an avulsion fracture from either the second MT base or the medial cuneiform, due to forceful abduction of the forefoot that avulses the Lisfranc ligament between the base of the second MT and the medial cuneiform – as can be seen in this case. On the AP view, the distance between the first and second metatarsals should be less than 2–3 mm. A normal lateral radiographic view of the foot should show the superior border of the first MT base lining up with the superior border of the medial cuneiform. If the dorsal surface of the proximal second MT is higher than the dorsal surface of the middle cuneiform then this is indicative of an injury. On a medial 30-degree oblique view of the foot, the cuboid should align with the medial border of the fourth MT.

MRI is accurate for detecting traumatic injury of the Lisfranc ligament and for predicting Lisfranc joint complex instability. Finally, with an ankle block or intravenous sedation, stress the foot under fluoroscopic examination with pressure on the medial forefoot, pushing laterally while the hindfoot is pushed medially. An AP view of the TMT joints reveals any significant instability.

Non-surgical management should be limited to patients who do not have fractures, or who have fractures that are undisplaced and stable under stress. If the clinical evaluation indicates the probability of a mild or moderate sprain and the radiograph shows no diastasis, then immobilization is suggested. Note the anterior tibial tendon can block reduction of a lateral Lisfranc dislocation; similarly, the peroneus brevis tendon can block a medial dislocation reduction. Combined closed reduction and casting has no role in the treatment of unstable injuries. All injuries that are displaced and unstable require surgery. A displacement of more than 2 mm requires open reduction and internal fixation. All

Lisfranc injuries that cannot be reduced and be made to remain stable by closed means should undergo internal fixation.

 KEY POINTS

- The Lisfranc joint is the articulation between the midfoot and forefoot.
- Radiological assessment involves AP, lateral and oblique views of the foot.
- Injury to the Lisfranc ligament can result in functional instability with loss of longitudinal and transverse arches.
- A diastasis greater than 2–3 mm between the base of the first and second metatarsals suggests a Lisfranc injury.
- The fleck sign seen on the AP radiograph is pathognomonic for a Lisfranc injury.
- Displacement of more than 2 mm requires open reduction and internal fixation.

CASE 43: A DEFORMED, SWOLLEN AND ULCERATED FOOT

History

A 55-year-old man has had insulin-dependent diabetes and been overweight for 10 years. He presents to his general practitioner about his left foot because he has noticed a moderate deformity and a significant amount of swelling. His wife has noticed also that the foot appears flatter when her husband is standing.

Examination

There is an area of ulceration on the sole of this man's left foot. There are signs also of inflammation including swelling, erythema and an increase in temperature of the skin compared to the unaffected foot (Figs. 43.1 and 43.2). On testing, there is no protective sensation.

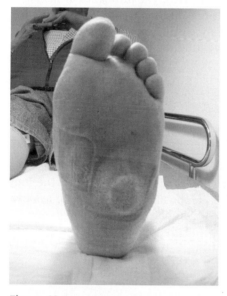

Figure 43.1   Figure 43.2

Questions

- What is the diagnosis?
- Who is at risk of this condition?
- How would you manage this condition?
- When is surgery indicated?

ANSWER 43

The diagnosis is a Charcot (neuropathic) joint, where damage has occurred through the lack of pain sensation to prevent damage. Charcot arthropathy results in progressive destruction of bone and soft tissues at weight-bearing joints. In its most severe form it may cause significant disruption of the bony architecture, including joint dislocations and fractures. Charcot arthropathy can occur at any joint but most commonly affects the lower regions: the foot and ankle. Bilateral disease occurs in fewer than 10 per cent of patients.

Any condition that leads to a sensory or autonomic neuropathy can cause a Charcot joint. Charcot arthropathy can occur as a complication of diabetes, syphilis, alcoholism, leprosy, meningomyleocele, spinal cord injury, syringomyelia, renal dialysis and congenital insensitivity to pain.

In the majority of cases, non-operative methods are preferred. The principles of management are to provide immobilization of the affected joint and reduce any areas of stress on the skin. Immobilization is usually accomplished by casting. Total-contact casts have been shown to allow patients to ambulate while preventing the progression of deformity. Casts must be checked weekly, and they should be replaced every 1–2 weeks. Patients with concomitant ulceration must have their casts changed weekly for ulcer evaluation and debridement. Serial plain radiographs should be taken approximately every month during the acute phase. Casting is usually necessary for 3–6 months and is discontinued based on clinical and radiographic assessments, and dermal temperature and signs of quiescence.

Surgery is uncommonly indicated for a Charcot foot when non-surgical methods fail: in particular when the deformity places the foot at risk of ulceration or when the foot can no longer be protected in accommodative footwear. The aim of surgery is to achieve a stable foot and ankle joint, maintaining the plantigrade position. The foot should be able to tolerate accommodative footwear and support ambulation of the patient. A major contraindication to surgery is active inflammation.

KEY POINTS

- Charcot arthropathy results in progressive destruction of bone and soft tissues at weight-bearing joints.
- Non-operative methods are the treatment of choice.
- The aim of surgery is to achieve a stable foot and ankle joint, maintaining the plantigrade position.

CASE 44: A STIFF SHOULDER

History

A 45-year-old woman was walking on a frosty morning when she slipped on a frozen path and landed on her right shoulder. She developed a persistent severe aching in her shoulder and later attended the emergency department. Investigations including an X-ray showed no fracture and she was reassured. A few days later she is still having difficulty washing and dressing, although there is hardly any pain in her shoulder. She has a medical history of diabetes but is otherwise fit and well.

Examination

This woman's shoulder area has no signs of obvious swelling or bruising. On palpation she has no tenderness or obvious deformity. She does, however, have a markedly reduced range of movement, particularly with external rotation. There are no associated neurological or vascular deficits. Radiographs of the shoulder are normal with no evidence of a fracture or avascular necrosis of the humeral head.

Questions

- What is the likely diagnosis?
- What are the three stages of this disease?
- Who is at increased risk of developing this condition?
- How would you manage this patient?

ANSWER 44

The diagnosis is a 'frozen shoulder', characterized by a global reduction in the range of movement and normal X-rays. This term was introduced by Codman in 1934. He described a painful shoulder condition of insidious onset that was associated with stiffness and difficulty sleeping on the affected side. Codman also identified the marked reduction in forward elevation and external rotation that are the hallmarks of the disease. In 1945, Naviesar coined the term 'adhesive capsulitis'.

Frozen shoulder typically has three phases: the painful phase, the stiffening phase and the thawing phase. During the initial phase there is a gradual onset of diffuse shoulder pain lasting from weeks to months. The stiffening phase is characterized by a progressive loss of motion that may last up to a year. The majority of patients lose glenohumeral external rotation, internal rotation and abduction during this phase. The final, thawing phase ranges from weeks to months and constitutes a period of gradual motion improvement. Once in this phase, the patient may require up to 9 months to regain a fully functional range of motion.

There is a higher incidence of frozen shoulder in patients with diabetes compared with the general population. The incidence among patients with insulin-dependent diabetes is even higher, with an increased frequency of bilateral frozen shoulder. Adhesive capsulitis has also been reported in patients with hyperthyroidism, ischaemic heart disease, and cervical spondylosis.

Non-steroidal anti-inflammatory drugs (NSAIDs) are recommended in the initial treatment phase. On reducing the inflammation and pain, the patient should be able to tolerate physical therapy. A subgroup of patients with frozen shoulder syndrome often fail to improve despite conservative measures. In these cases, interventions such as manipulation, distension arthrography or open surgical release may be beneficial.

 KEY POINTS

- Frozen shoulder (adhesive capsulitis) is a painful shoulder condition of insidious onset with stiffness.
- There are three phases: painful, stiffening and thawing.
- The incidence is raised in diabetics.
- The majority of cases resolve with conservative management.

CASE 45: ELBOW PAIN (1)

History

A 40-year-old right-handed mechanic has been working long days and starts to develop pain in the lateral aspect of his right elbow. The pain is worst when he is at work and it is affecting his ability to work properly, so he goes to see his general practitioner.

Examination

This man's pain is localized to the lateral epicondyle of his elbow. There is no obvious swelling or deformity. On palpation there is a point of maximal tenderness just distal to the lateral epicondyle. Wrist extension and supination against resistance produces pain. His pain is reproduced on extension/flexion of his affected wrist.

Questions

- What is the diagnosis?
- What further investigations are commonly undertaken in this condition?
- What are the management options?

ANSWER 45

The diagnosis is work-related lateral epicondylitis (commonly called 'tennis elbow'). It is an overuse injury involving the extensor muscles that originate on the lateral epicondylar region of the distal humerus. It is more properly termed a tendinosis that specifically involves the origin of the extensor carpi radialis brevis muscle. Histologically, the tendons are invaded with vascular granulation tissue and fibroblasts. There is notable absence of inflammatory cells in the affected area.

Any activity involving wrist extension and/or supination can be associated with overuse of the muscles originating at the lateral epicondyle. Tennis has been the activity most commonly associated with the disorder. For work-related lateral epicondylitis, a systematic review identified three risk factors: handling tools heavier than 1 kg, handling loads heavier than 20 kg at least ten times per day, and repetitive movements for more than two hours per day

X-rays of the affected elbow are usually normal but in chronic cases can show calcification of the origin of the affected tendon (extensor carpi radialis brevis, ECRB). MRI is helpful to exclude any ligamentous or tendinous injury to the elbow. Also, MRI can help confirm the presence of degenerative tissue in the ECRB origin. Ultrasonography of the elbow is a reasonable alternative to MRI if expertise is available.

Anaesthetic injections into the origin of the extensor carpi radialis brevis can help confirm the diagnosis, as the patient should experience relief from symptoms.

Up to 95 per cent of patients with tennis elbow respond to conservative measures. The goal is cessation of the offending activity. Rest, use of a counterforce brace, and non-steroidal anti-inflammatory drugs (NSAIDs) often provide relief. Often, wrist splinting is necessary. Both corticosteroid and autologous blood injections have been shown to be effective. Corticosteroid injections at the lateral epicondyle have been shown to significantly decrease pain and would be recommended in the present case of an active worker.

When the patient is free of pain through a full range of motion, begin strengthening therapy in a very slow and progressive way. When the patient regains strength and resumption of activity, place the emphasis of treatment on preventing future irritation.

If the present case were unresponsive to conservative therapy over 6 months (including corticosteroid injections), he would be eligible for surgery. Most surgical procedures involve debridement of the diseased tissue of the extensor carpi radialis brevis muscle with decortication of the lateral epicondyle. This procedure can be performed through open, percutaneous and arthroscopic approaches.

 KEY POINTS

- Tennis elbow involves the origin of the extensor carpi radialis brevis muscle.
- Any activity involving wrist extension and/or supination can be associated with this condition.
- X-rays are usually normal but can show calcification of the affected tendon. MRI or ultrasonography are useful investigations in this condition.
- Anaesthetic injections into the origin of the ECRB muscle can help confirm the diagnosis.
- Most patients respond to conservative management.

CASE 46: ELBOW PAIN (2)

History

A 25-year-old vintage-car mechanic has been extremely busy preparing a fleet of cars for an exhibition. He has developed severe pain over the medial aspect of his right elbow which is limiting his ability to work, so he visits his general practitioner. He reports that this is not the first time this pain has occurred.

Examination

This young man's pain is localized to the medial epicondyle of his right elbow. He has tenderness to palpation over the anterior aspect of the medial epicondyle. There is no obvious swelling or deformity of the elbow and no muscle wasting. Elbow range of movement and neurovascular examination are normal. Pain over the medial epicondyle is aggravated with resisted wrist flexion and pronation.

Questions

- What is the diagnosis?
- What further examinations and investigations are commonly undertaken in this condition?
- What are the management options?

ANSWER 46

The diagnosis is medial epicondylitis (commonly called 'golfer's elbow'). It typically presents with pain on the medial aspect of the elbow associated with an exacerbation of pain in resisted wrist flexion. This condition was first described in 1882 by Henry J. Morris and is classified as an overuse syndrome. The flexor carpi radialis and the pronator teres are commonly involved at the insertion of the medial epicondyle; the muscles less commonly involved are the palmaris longus, the flexor digitorum superficialis, and the flexor carpi ulnaris.

This condition is seen most commonly in sports involving repetitive valgus stress, flexion and pronation, such as occurs in golf and baseball. Ulnar neuropathy may be associated in approximately half of cases. Magnetic resonance images and histology show the presence of micro-tears in the flexor–pronator tendons without inflammation. Medial epicondylitis is more common in men and the peak incidences are in the third and fifth decades of life.

X-rays of the affected elbow are usually normal but can show calcification at the affected tendon's origin. MRI is sensitive and specific in the evaluation of medial epicondylitis. This modality allows assessment of the tendons, ulnar nerve and medial collateral ligament. For confirmation of the diagnosis, a local anaesthetic can be injected into the medial epicondyle over the area of maximal tenderness; complete relief of pain should be expected.

In the majority of cases, conservative management works and should be the initial treatment. The first step is to identify and restrict the activities that cause the pain. Changes in working conditions or sporting activities can help. Non-steroidal anti-inflammatory drugs (NSAIDs), physical therapy and an epicondylar band over the forearm muscles to reduce force transmission to the tendons are helpful. Return to regular activities should be progressive to minimize the chances of recurrence. Steroid infiltration can be considered after failed conservative management. Surgery is considered if conservative measures fail after 6–12 months. It involves release of the muscle group origin from the tendon.

 KEY POINTS

- Flexor carpi radialis and the pronator teres are commonly involved in golfer's elbow.
- The mechanism is through repetitive valgus stress, flexion and pronation.
- X-rays are usually normal. MRI is sensitive and specific in the evaluation.
- An injection of local anaesthetic is a useful diagnostic test.

CASE 47: A PAINFUL WRIST

History

A 50-year-old woman working as a medical secretary has been involved with converting a paper records system to an electronic system. She has been lifting and carrying a lot of heavy boxes of files as part of this. Now she has developed progressive pain in the dorsal/radial aspect of the base of her right wrist and radial styloid.

Examination

This woman has swelling over the dorsoradial aspect of her left wrist. On palpation, she has some palpable thickening in the same region and tenderness over the styloid process of the distal radius. When the patient is asked to make a fist over the thumb and ulna deviate the wrist (Fig. 47.1), she reports increased pain in the region of the radial styloid. She has no neurological or vascular deficits.

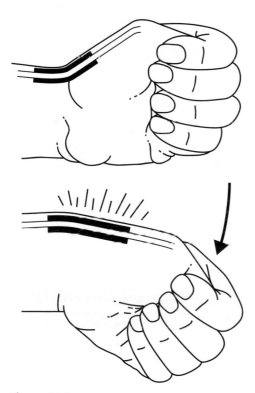

Figure 47.1

Questions

- What is the diagnosis, and how would you confirm it?
- What is the differential diagnosis?
- What do you know about the pathology of this condition?
- How would you manage this patient?

ANSWER 47

This condition is called De Quervain's tenosynovitis, first described in 1895. It is characterized by a history of repetitive strain, and dorsoradial pain exacerbated by ulna deviation of the wrist. There is reactive thickening of the sheath around the first extensor compartment of the wrist. The tendons of the abductor pollicis longus and the extensor pollicis brevis pass through the first dorsal compartment. The first dorsal compartment over the radial styloid becomes thickened and feels bone hard; the area becomes tender. The exact cause of this problem is not clear. Overuse can initiate it, but it can occur spontaneously, particularly in middle-aged women and sometimes during pregnancy.

The classic manoeuvre to diagnose this condition is achieved using the Finkelstein test. This involves making a fist over the thumb and moving the wrist into ulna deviation, as shown in Fig. 47.1. The pain is reproduced in the region of the radial styloid.

The differential diagnosis includes the following.

- Arthritis at the base of the thumb. The grind test will be negative in DeQuervain's but positive in degenerative joint disease affecting the carpometacarpal (CMC) joint. The grind test is performed by pushing the thumb against the CMC joint while also rotating it to produce a grinding-type motion. If in doubt, radiographs of the first CMC joint may reveal degenerative changes.
- Intersection syndrome. This can arise if the tendons of the first wrist compartment cross over the tendons of the second compartment just proximal to the extensor retinaculum. This causes irritation between the tendons just proximal to the wrist joint.
- Wartenberg's syndrome. This is an isolated neuritis of the superficial radial nerve. These patients have a positive Tinel sign and complain of pain over the dorsoradial aspect of the wrist.

Conservative management initially involves a thumb spica splint, or a cast for a month with a steroid injection into the first extensor compartment sheath. Surgical release of the first extensor tendon sheath with synovectomy is considered for persistent or recurrent De Quervains's disease. Ensure that the abductor pollicis longus and the extensor pollicis brevis are released.

 KEY POINTS

- De Quervain's tenosynovitis involves reactive thickening of the sheath around the first extensor compartment of the wrist. The tendons affected are abductor pollicis longus and the extensor pollicis brevis.
- A positive Finkelstein test helps to confirm the diagnosis.
- Initial management involves a splint plus a steroid injection. Surgical treatment in persistent or recurrent cases involves release of the first extensor tendon sheath.

CASE 48: A DEFORMED FINGER

History

A 55-year-old woman with diabetes was trying to do some knitting when she noticed that one of her right fingers was painful and intermittently stiff. She went to see her general practitioner for an explanation. She has no history of trauma. She reports she has difficulty achieving a full range of movement of the finger and complains of painful clicking of the finger when she tries to make a fist.

Examination

This woman's finger remains flexed at the proximal interphalangeal (PIP) joint even when she tries to unclench her fist (Fig. 48.1), but with further effort the finger suddenly extends fully with a snap. At the level of the distal palmar crease she has a nodule that is tender to palpation over the metacarpophalangeal (MCP) joint. On attempting to straighten the affected finger, a painful click is elicited when the finger is fully extended.

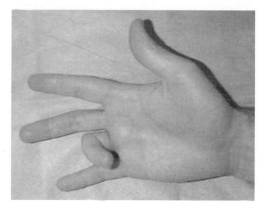

Figure 48.1

Questions:

- What is the diagnosis?
- How would you manage this condition?

ANSWER 48

The diagnosis is 'trigger finger', a name chosen because typically the finger suddenly extends fully with a snap. It results from thickening of the flexor tendon within the distal aspect of the palm. The gliding of the flexor tendon within the tendon sheath is affected. This results in abrupt flexion of the finger. There is often tenderness over the A1 pulley (a fibrous structure located at the MCP joint through which the flexor tendon passes) and intermittent restriction to flexion and extension of the finger. A nodule may develop on the tendon causing the tendon to get stuck in the pulley when attempting to extend the digit. Trigger digits are most commonly seen in adults aged between 50 and 60 years, and less commonly can be seen in congenital cases affecting the thumb in children.

In the majority of cases a steroid infiltration into the affected tendon sheath can give symptomatic relief. Splinting of the finger can help in reducing inflammation. Digits that fail to respond to two or three injections may benefit from surgery. Surgical release of the A1 flexor pulley will allow the inflamed tendon to pass through and relieve symptoms. Congenital cases do not respond to injections and require surgical intervention.

 KEY POINTS

- Gliding of the flexor tendon within the tendon sheath is affected in trigger finger.
- Often there is tenderness over the A1 pulley. A nodule may develop on the tendon, causing the tendon to get stuck in the pulley.
- A steroid infiltration into the affected tendon sheath can give symptomatic relief in the majority of cases. Digits that fail to respond to 2–3 injections may benefit from surgical release of the A1 pulley.

CASE 49: A PAINLESS CONTRACTURE DEFORMITY OF A HAND

History

A 50-year-old gardener was keen on working in his garden but commented to his wife that he was suffering from increasing problems with his hands. They noticed that his right hand had some thickening in the palm associated with some skin puckering, and he could not fully straighten his fingers (Fig. 49.1). They decided that he should visit their general practitioner. He has a medical history of epilepsy.

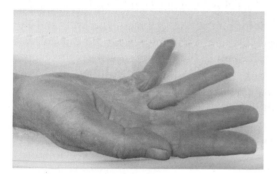

Figure 49.1

Examination

As noticed by the patient, there is thickening in the palm and some skin puckering, and he cannot fully straighten his fingers. He is able to make a full fist but unable to straighten his hand flat on the table. In addition he has evidence of dorsal knuckle pads in the affected hand.

Questions

- What is the diagnosis?
- What is the pathology of this condition?
- What are the signs of aggressive disease?
- How would you manage this patient?

ANSWER 49

This man has Dupuytren's disease of the palmar fascia, first described by Baron Guillaume Dupuytren (1777–1835). The condition can be inherited as an autosomal dominant trait. The clinical features are nodular thickening in the palm, with flexion contractures at the metacarpophalangeal (MCP) and proximal interphalangeal (PIP) joints as show in Fig. 49.1. Dorsal knuckle pads may be thickened (Garrod's pad) and both hands may be involved. Typically it is painless.

Dupuytren's contracture is a benign, slowly progressive fibroproliferative disease of the palmar fascia. After the initial proliferative phase the fibrous tissue and fascial bands within the fingers contract causing flexion deformity of the fingers at the MCP and PIP joints, and rarely the distal (DIP) joint. The MCP joint contracture may be caused by a pretendinous cord or by contracture of the spiral band. PIP joint contractures are caused by the central and spiral cords and the thumb may show a flexion deformity. Abduction may be limited in the fingers as the natatory ligament becomes contracted. The disease presents most commonly in the ring and little fingers and is bilateral in 45 per cent of cases. The fibrous attachment to the skin causes the puckering. Similar nodules may be seen on the sole of the foot (Ledderhose disease) and in fibrosis of the corpus cavernosum (Peyronie disease).

A more aggressive form of the disease is associated with a positive family history, onset before the age of 40 years, bilateral involvement, involvement of the radial digits and ectopic disease (feet and penis).

Dupuytren's disease is more common in males and people of northern European origin. It can be associated with prior hand trauma, alcoholic cirrhosis, epilepsy (due to medications such as phenytoin) and diabetes. The prevalence increases with age.

Mild cases may not need any treatment. Surgery is indicated in progressive contractures and established deformity – as in this case. Surgical excision of the diseased fascia (fasciectomy) is the treatment of choice. Recurrence or extension of the disease after operation is not uncommon, particularly in patients with associated fibrosis (Ledderhose and Peyronie). Surgery is generally indicated for MCP joint contractures of 20–30 degrees. Any degree of flexion contracture of the PIP joint is an indication for surgery. The operation will involve either a fasciotomy (incising the fascia only), fasciectomy (removing as much fascia as possible), dermofasciectomy (removing the diseased fascia and overlying skin), or regional fasciectomy (excising only the involved fascia).

 KEY POINTS

- Dupuytren's contracture is a slowly progressive fibroproliferative disease of the palmar fascia. It presents most commonly in the ring and little fingers.
- Look for nodular thickening in the palm, flexion contractures at the MCP and PIP joints, and Garrod's pad.
- It is associated with prior hand trauma, alcoholic cirrhosis, epilepsy (due to medications such as phenytoin) and diabetes.
- Surgery is indicated in progressive contracture and established deformity.

CASE 50: A PAINFUL WRIST FOLLOWING A FALL

History

A 26-year-old carpenter slipped on a wet floor and landed on his left hand. He immediately felt some wrist pain. The pain did not improve by the following day and prevented him from working, so he visited the emergency department. He is otherwise fit and well. He smokes about one pack of cigarettes per day.

Examination

This young man has some swelling in the anatomical snuffbox, associated with some palpable tenderness in the area. The pain is aggravated when the thumb or wrist is moved and when the man tries to grip objects. Radiographs are shown in Fig. 50.1.

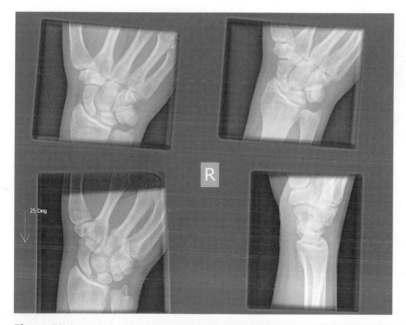

Figure 50.1

Questions
- What is the diagnosis?
- Describe any special clinical provocative tests.
- What are the anatomical features of this area, and its blood supply?
- How would you further investigate this patient to confirm the diagnosis?
- What complications can you predict?

ANSWER 50

The diagnosis is a scaphoid fracture. This diagnosis is more likely in the presence of tenderness to palpation in the anatomical snuffbox and on the volar scaphoid tubercle. A special provocative manoeuvre is known as the Watson (scaphoid shift) test. Place the patients' wrist into full ulna deviation and extension. Press the patient's thumb with his other hand and move the wrist into radial deviation and flexion. If the scaphoid and lunate are unstable, the dorsal pole of the scaphoid subluxes over the dorsal rim of the radius and the patient complains of pain – indicating a positive test.

The scaphoid is the most commonly fractured carpal bone, being involved in up to 75 per cent of all carpal fractures. Scaphoid waist fractures are the most common type (65 per cent), followed by proximal pole fractures (30 per cent). Scaphoid fractures are uncommon in children because the physis of the distal radius usually fails first. In elderly patients, the distal radial metaphysis usually fails before the scaphoid can fracture.

The scaphoid is an irregularly shaped bone of which 80 per cent is covered by articular cartilage. The scaphoid flexes with wrist flexion and radial deviation and it extends during wrist extension and ulnar deviation. Anatomically, the scaphoid is divided into proximal, middle (termed the waist) and distal thirds. Most of the blood supply to the scaphoid enters distally. The proximal part of the scaphoid has no blood vessels entering it, depending instead on vessels that pierce the mid-portion in a retrograde direction, thereby placing the proximal pole at increased risk of avascular necrosis when fractured.

Scaphoid X-rays preferably include a posteroanterior (PA) view, a true lateral view, an oblique view, and a PA ulnar-deviated view. The PA in ulnar deviation allows viewing of the scaphoid in extension, while the lateral view allows an evaluation of instability. When the scaphoid is destabilized via ligament disruption or fracture, the lunate and triquetrum may excessively dorsiflex and yield a dorsal intercalary segment instability (DISI) deformity. Occasionally, a fractured scaphoid is not visible on the initial radiographs. In such cases, a repeat X-ray in 10–14 days may reveal a fracture line after some resorption. If a diagnosis still cannot be confirmed with confidence on routine films, MRI of the wrist is recommended. While CT scanning is useful in assessing union, fractures with less than 1 mm of displacement are often not detected.

Non-union is not uncommon as a complication after scaphoid fractures because the blood supply to this bone is poor. Smokers have a higher incidence of non-union. Occasionally, the blood supply is poor enough to lead to avascular necrosis. If non-union is not detected, subsequent arthritis in the wrist can develop. Imaging using a combination of plain X-rays, MRI and/or CT can help confirm a non-union and avascular necrosis. If the scaphoid fails to unite, consider a bone graft. A graft can be harvested locally from the same forearm or from the iliac crest. Sometimes it is necessary to use a bone graft with its own blood supply (a vascularized graft).

 KEY POINTS

- Scaphoid waist fractures are the most common type (65 per cent), followed by proximal pole fractures.
- Clinical examination reveals tenderness in the anatomical snuffbox.
- A special test is Watson's provocative manoeuvre.
- Treatment is with a scaphoid cast.
- Proximal pole fractures often require surgery and they have a high non-union rate.

CASE 51: A SWOLLEN JOINT AND FEVER

History

An 84-year-old woman with diabetes has been admitted to the emergency department with an acutely swollen and painful left knee. She has been unwell with a raised temperature and productive cough for the last week and for the last 24 hours has been unable to bear weight because of her knee pain.

Examination

This elderly woman is unwell, sweaty and febrile. Her pulse is 108 bpm and blood pressure 98/60 mmHg. Oxygen saturation on room air is 92 per cent. Her left knee is held rigid in fixed flexion and is hot and red with a moderate effusion. Her respiratory rate is 22/min. There is decreased expansion on the right side, with dullness to percussion, increased vocal resonance and coarse crackles at the base. The remainder of her examination is normal.

INVESTIGATIONS		
		Normal range
Haemoglobin	14.2 g/dL	13.3–17.7 g/dL
White cell count	18.3×10^9/L	$3.9–10.6 \times 10^9$/L
Platelets	542×10^9/L	$150–440 \times 10^9$/L
ESR	45 mm/h	<10 mm/h
CRP	>160 mg/L	<5 mg/L
Chest X-ray	Right basal consolidation	

Questions

- What is the diagnosis and likely explanation for the right knee pain and swelling?
- What is the immediate further investigation and management?

ANSWER 51

This elderly woman's diagnosis is bronchopneumonia with a septic arthritis. Septic arthritis is an orthopaedic emergency. This patient is already tachycardic, hypotensive and hypoxic and needs prompt assessment, diagnosis and management by medical and surgical teams. The diagnosis hinges on the detection of bacteria in the synovial fluid, and a joint aspiration with microbiological evaluation of the aspirate is critical.

Patients with septic arthritis are typically unwell with fevers and malaise and the joint pain is severe. Risk factors for the development of septic arthritis are:

- abnormal, damaged or prosthetic joints
- concurrent or recent bacterial infection
- immunocompromise
- extremes of age.

The patient presented here has several clearly identifiable risk factors: current infection, relative immunocompromise in the form of diabetes, and advanced age.

Septic arthritis is divided into non-gonococcal (80 per cent of cases) and gonococcal disease. Within non-gonococcal septic arthritis, the most common organisms isolated are *Staphylococcus*, *Streptococcus* and Gram-negative bacilli. These causative organisms reach the joint through direct inoculation, spread from neighbouring infected tissue (e.g. osteomyelitis, cellulitis) or haematogenous spread during bacteraemia, which is the likely scenario in this case. Gonococcal disease occurs in sexually active groups and tends to present with a more polyarticular, migratory pattern, tenosynovitis and a rash; the precipitating infection may be asymptomatic, particularly in women. It can be hard to diagnose as even synovial fluid cultures have a low positive yield, with up to 75 per cent of cultures being negative. It is also important to remember that gonococcal arthritis is not the same as reactive arthritis following genitourinary infection; the latter is an inflammatory reaction to extra-articular infection and is often managed with local intra-articular steroid injections.

The treatment of choice in septic arthritis is antibiotic therapy which should be commenced as soon as possible. In the absence of definitive culture results, the best initial choice would be a broad-spectrum antibiotic with activity against the most likely culprits (such as a second-generation cephalosporin). Antimicrobial therapy can then be adjusted according to culture results and sensitivities. Cartilage is highly susceptible to damage from infected synovial fluid, so a surgical washout may be required, particularly if the hip is involved. Antibiotic therapy should be continued for 4–6 weeks.

 KEY POINTS

- Any acutely hot or painful joint is septic arthritis until proven otherwise.
- Investigation of choice is aspiration of the joint fluid and microbiological assessment.
- In likely cases of septic arthritis, commence antibiotic therapy as soon as possible.

CASE 52: PAINFUL HANDS IN A YOUNG WOMAN

History

A 34-year-old woman attends the rheumatology outpatient clinic with a 6-month history of painful hands. Previously fit and well, she developed mild pain in her metacarpophalangeal (MCP) joints which deteriorated over a few weeks to profound pain and marked stiffness affecting both hands and wrists, particularly in the morning. Her symptoms are now very intrusive. Her general practitioner has prescribed diclofenac with minimal benefit. She is otherwise well but is becoming isolated and depressed; she delayed going to see her GP because she was concerned that she had developed the same 'rheumatism' as her grandmother who was wheelchair-dependent.

Examination

This woman is thin and tearful. She has marked soft-tissue swelling of her wrists, MCPs and several proximal interphalangeal (PIP) joints in both her hands, and has reduced grip strength bilaterally. Apart from a non-tender nodule on her elbow, the rest of her examination is entirely normal. A radiograph is shown in Fig. 52.1.

🔍 INVESTIGATIONS

		Normal range
Haemoglobin	10.9 g/dL	13.3–17.7 g/dL
Mean corpuscular volume (MCV)	85 fL	80–99 fL
White cell count	7.4×10^9/L	$3.9–10.6 \times 10^9$/L
Platelets	523×10^9/L	$150–440 \times 10^9$/L
ESR	62 mm/h	<10 mm/h
CRP	94 mg/L	<5 mg/L
Rheumatoid factor (RF)	Positive	
Anti-citrullinated peptide antibody (ACPA)	Positive	
Anti-nuclear factor (ANA)	Negative	

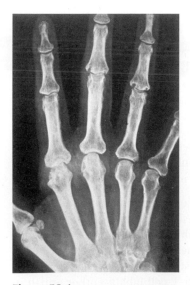

Figure 52.1

Questions

- What is the most likely diagnosis?
- What other possibilities are there?
- How would you manage this patient?

ANSWER 52

The diagnosis is rheumatoid arthritis (RA), the most common of the inflammatory arthropathies. Her symptoms of early-morning stiffness and pain, combined with soft-tissue rather than bony swelling, are classic patterns for inflammatory disease. Although, as in this case, RA affects principally the small joints of the hands (and feet), it may progress to involve any synovial joint and may be complicated by extra-articular features (see below). Her possible family history for RA is not unusual due to the presence of susceptibility genes such as HLA-DR.

The thrombocytosis, elevated inflammatory markers and normocytic anaemia seen here are very common in patients with active disease. Rheumatoid factor, a self-reactive IgG, is detected in up to 70 per cent of RA patients, and the presence of rheumatoid nodules on examination indicates such seropositivity and a worse prognosis. RF has relatively low specificity and is found in other inflammatory conditions (e.g. Sjögren's syndrome, cryoglobulinaemia), certain infections and apparently healthy individuals. ACPA, however, offers a greater specificity and may become positive before the development of symptoms. The X-ray of her hand reveals many of the cardinal features of established RA: soft-tissue swelling, periarticular osteopenia, joint space narrowing and bony erosions (in this case particularly affecting the third and fourth PIPs). There is also evidence of joint destruction and ankylosis in the carpal bones.

> **!** **Major differential diagnoses for small-joint arthropathy**
>
> - Rheumatoid arthritis
> - Psoriatic arthritis in association with skin and typically nail disease
> - Post-infective arthritis following streptococcal or viral infection
> - Systemic lupus erythematosus (SLE) in the presence of pronounced extra-articular symptoms and a positive ANA
> - Parvovirus arthropathy, particularly in those with contact with small children

Parvovirus arthropathy is classically short-lived (<6 weeks), with normal radiology and immunology (beyond IgM antibodies to parvovirus).

Treatment of RA involves a multidisciplinary team (MDT). Specialist nurses, occupational therapists and physiotherapists are invaluable sources of support, advice, education and treatment and this patient should be referred immediately. Medical therapy focuses on disease-modifying anti-rheumatic drugs (DMARDs) such as methotrexate, sulphasalazine, leflunomide and hydroxychloroquine which may be used individually or in combination. Many are contraindicated in pregnancy and breast-feeding and this should be specifically discussed as the patient is of child-bearing age. DMARD therapy also necessitates regular blood monitoring as many are potentially myelosuppressive or hepatotoxic. All DMARDs take up to 3 months to have full clinical effect, so she should be offered an intramuscular injection of steroid as immediate treatment for her acute inflammatory symptoms.

If she fails to respond to standard DMARDs, 'biologic' (i.e. monoclonal antibody) treatment against pathogenic cytokines or cells could be used. The most common biologic agent is anti-TNF-α; infliximab, adalimumab, golimumab and certolizumab are monoclonal antibodies directed against the TNF-α molecule, whereas etanercept is an Fc fusion protein and acts as a 'decoy' receptor for TNF-α. If she still suffers from active disease despite anti-TNF-α treatment, anti-B-cell (rituximab), anti-T-cell (abatacept) or anti-IL-6 receptor (tocilizumab) therapy are alternative therapeutic options.

! ACR/EULAR classification criteria for rheumatoid arthritis (2010)*

Clinical finding	Score
Joint involvement with clinical synovitis	(0–5)
1 large joint**	0
2–10 large joints	1
1–3 small joints (± large joint involvement)***	2
4–10 small joints (± large joint involvement)	3
>10 joints (with at least one small joint)	5
Serology	(0–3)
Negative RF and negative ACPA	0
Low positive RF or low positive ACPA	2
High positive RF or high positive ACPA	3
Acute-phase reactants	(0–1)
Normal CRP and normal ESR	0
Abnormal CRP or abnormal ESR	1
Duration of symptoms	(0–1)
< 6 weeks	0
≥ 6 weeks	1

* To be classified with rheumatoid arthritis, a patient must score at least 6 points.
** Large joints are ankles, elbows, shoulders, hips and knees.
*** Small joints are wrists and small joints of the hands and feet.

! Extra-articular features of rheumatoid arthritis

Systemic	*Ocular*	*Respiratory*
Malaise	(Epi)scleritis	Pulmonary nodules
Fatigue	Anterior uveitis	Interstitial lung disease
Weight loss	Keratoconjunctivitis sicca	Pleural effusion
		Bronchiolitis obliterans
Cardiac	*Renal*	*Haematological*
Accelerated atheroma	Amyloid	Anaemia
Conduction defects	NSAID-induced nephropathy	Thrombocytosis
Coronary vasculitis		Felty's syndrome
Pericarditis		
Neurological	*Dermatological*	
Compression neuropathy	Vasculitis	
Mononeuritis multiplex	Palmar erythema	

🔑 KEY POINTS

- Early morning stiffness is a cardinal feature of inflammatory disease.
- Not all patients with RA have rheumatoid factor (RF), and not all patients with RF have RA; ACPA has greater specificity for RA than rheumatoid factor.
- Always consider parvovirus arthropathy in a young patient with small-joint arthritis.
- All DMARDs have a lag effect and require close monitoring.

CASE 53: BACK PAIN IN A YOUNG MAN

History

A 26-year-old man presents with a 6-month history of back and buttock pain and stiff-ness. His symptoms localize to his lumbar spine and right buttock and are particularly marked first thing in the morning, but start to settle within a couple of hours. The pain never spreads down the back of the leg and he has not noticed any change in sensation or loss of power. He is otherwise fit and well, with the exception of two episodes of an acutely painful red eye for which he received 'eye drops' from the ophthalmology service. He is self-employed with two children and smokes heavily.

Examination

This young man has dramatically reduced lumbar spinal movements in all planes but cervical movements are full and pain-free. His right hip is irritable with reduced range of movement, particularly external rotation. There is a small effusion of the left knee with evidence of Achilles tendinopathy and plantar fasciitis on the left foot. The remainder of his examination is normal. MRI of the lumbosacral spine and sacroiliac joints are shown in Figs 53.1 and 53.2.

INVESTIGATIONS		
		Normal range
Haemoglobin	15.2 g/dL	13.3–17.7 g/dL
White cell count	5.6×10^9/L	$3.9–10.6 \times 10^9$/L
Platelets	329×10^9/L	$150–440 \times 10^9$/L
ESR	38 mm/h	<10 mm/h
CRP	42 mg/L	<5 mg/L
HLA-B27	Positive	

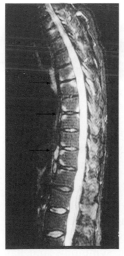

Figure 53.1

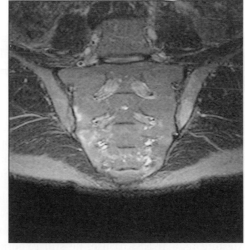

Figure 53.2

Questions
* What is the most likely diagnosis?
* What does the MRI show?
* How would you manage this patient?

ANSWER 53

The patient's symptoms are a classic description of inflammatory spinal disease (spondylo-arthropathy) and sacroiliitis. In addition he has evidence of peripheral arthropathy, tendinopathy, possible extra-articular symptoms in the form of previous ocular disease, and an elevated inflammatory response. The most likely unifying cause of these symptoms and signs is ankylosing spondylitis (AS). The presence of the MHC molecule HLA-B27 is supportive but not diagnostic of this disease: although more than 95 per cent of patients with AS are B27-positive, up to 10 per cent of the normal population is also B27-positive in the absence of spinal disease.

> **! Major differential diagnoses of spondyloarthropathy**
>
> - Ankylosing spondylitis (prototypical spondyloarthritis), most common in males under 35 years of age
> - Psoriatic arthropathy
> - Enteropathic, associated with inflammatory bowel disease, but unrelated to disease activity
> - Reactive arthritis following genitourinary or gastrointestinal infection

Diagnostic confusion may be caused by overlapping symptom complexes between spondyloarthropathies (e.g. red eye, rash, gastrointestinal upset), and some patients do not fit neatly into one diagnostic category, being described as having undifferentiated spinal disease.

This patient's MRI highlights areas of high water content (joint inflammation and bone oedema) and shows typical features of AS: the corners of the lumbar vertebrae are 'shiny' with oedema and there is symmetrical inflammatory change at the sacroiliac joints with irregularity of the joint space. The inflammation leads to symptoms of pain and stiffness, while fibrosis and ossification at these sites generates signs of increasing spinal restriction. One such clinical measure of spinal restriction is Schober's index: two marks on the lumbar spine 15 cm apart (5 cm below and 10 cm above the posterior superior iliac spines) should increase to >20 cm apart on forward flexion; lateral spinal flexion and cervical neck movements should also be assessed regularly. In late-stage disease, patients may develop a 'question-mark' posture with loss of lumbar lordosis, exaggerated thoracic kyphosis and hyperextension at the neck. Complete spinal fusion (ankylosis) may occur and is surprisingly painless, unless microfractures develop due to spinal rigidity and concomitant osteoporosis.

Although AS is dominated by axial disease, large-joint peripheral arthropathy (hip and knee), enthesopathy and tendinopathy may also develop. Extra-articular features include anterior uveitis, which occurs in up to 40 per cent of patients (with no relation to spinal disease activity), apical pulmonary fibrosis and aortic regurgitation.

Treatment for AS focuses on physiotherapy and non-steroidal anti-inflammatory drugs (NSAIDs). In view of the risk of chest wall fusion following costochondritis or costovertebritis and possible restrictive lung disease, this patient must also be advised to give up smoking. If, despite regular NSAID use, he still experiences marked symptoms and has objective serological and/or radiological evidence of ongoing inflammatory disease, anti-TNF-α therapy is indicated.

| KEY POINTS |

- Ankylosing spondylitis is the most common cause of inflammatory spinal pain.
- HLA-B27 is not a diagnostic test.
- The investigation of choice is an MRI scan of the lumbosacral spine and sacroiliac joints.
- Treatment is physiotherapy, NSAIDs and anti-TNF-α in the presence of refractory disease.

CASE 54: CLUMSINESS

History

A 64-year-old man is referred urgently by his general practitioner with acute neuropathy. Two days prior to presentation the patient awoke to find himself unable to lift his right foot and toes while walking, such that he kept tripping. Over the next 24 hours he found he had lost control of his left thumb and could not grip things properly. His problems were associated with altered sensation in his hand and foot. His past medical history is entirely unremarkable.

Examination

This man has a high steppage gait and inability to dorsiflex the right foot and walk on his heels only. Sensation is also diminished over the top of the foot and ankle. In the left hand, there is loss of abduction and opposition of the thumb and reduced sensation in the lateral three and a half digits.

Questions
- What is the cause of these symptoms?
- What further investigations would be appropriate?

ANSWER 54

This patient has complete loss of median and common peroneal nerve function. The abruptness of the onset and anatomically distinct nature of the loss suggests an intrinsic nerve problem rather than a compressive neuropathy. The diagnosis is therefore mono-neuritis multiplex – the loss of motor and sensory function of multiple individual peripheral nerves. Mononeuritis multiplex arises due to interruption of the vasa nervorum, the blood supply to peripheral nerves, and one of the most common causes for this is vasculitis (another major cause is diabetes mellitus, but not relevant in this particular case).

Vasculitis – inflammation of blood vessels and subsequent obstruction to blood flow – can be primary (idiopathic) or secondary, in which case it is associated with an under-lying condition such as rheumatoid arthritis. Primary vasculitis is divided clinically according to the size of the vessel involved (see the box).

! **Clinical classification of idiopathic vasculitis**	
Large vessel	Giant cell (temporal) arteritis
	Takayasu's arteritis
Medium vessel	Polyarteritis nodosa
	Kawasaki's disease
Small vessel	Anti-neutrophil cytoplasmic antibody (ANCA) associated: Wegener's granulomatosis, microscopic polyangiitis
	Churg–Strauss syndrome (may be ANCA-positive)
	Immune-complex mediated
	Cryoglobulinaemic vasculitis: hypersensitivity vasculitis
	Henoch–Schönlein vasculitis

Mononeuritis multiplex can be caused by any of the medium or small vessel vasculitides and the patient should be approached with this differential in mind. Specific clinical features from each of the differential diagnoses should be sought in the history and examination, bearing in mind that there will be considerable overlap; skin involvement, for example, is very common in all types of vasculitis. More discriminating features would include:

- livedo reticularis, back pain, testicular pain in polyarteritis nodosa
- sinus or audiovestibular disease in Wegener's granulomatosis
- adult-onset asthma or nasal polyps in Churg–Strauss syndrome
- abdominal pain and rectal bleeding in Henoch–Schönlein vasculitis.

Investigations in patients with suspected vasculitis should be chosen to confirm the diagnosis and define the extent and severity of organ involvement. Many of the investi-gations listed in the box would be appropriate in this patient. A crucial investigation in cases of mononeuritis multiplex is nerve biopsy and a common site for this procedure is the sural nerve.

! Common investigations and results in a patient with suspected vasculitis	
Full blood count	Anaemia of chronic disease
	Thrombocytosis
	Eosinophilia (Churg–Strauss syndrome)
Renal function incl. urine dipstick	Assessment of renal involvement
ESR and CRP	Elevated
ANCA	cANCA commonly Wegener's granulomatosis
	pANCA commonly microscopic polyangiitis and Churg–Strauss
ANA	Negative in primary vasculitis, positive in SLE-induced disease
RF	Positive in cryoglobulinaemia and rheumatoid vasculitis
Complement	Low in SLE-induced vasculitis and cryoglobulinaemia
Cryoglobulins	Positive in cryoglobulinaemic vasculitis
Hepatitis serology	Hepatitis B associated with polyarteritis nodosa
	Hepatitis C associated with cryoglobulinaemia
HIV serology	May be positive in any vasculitis
Other (where indicated)	Chest X-ray (pulmonary disease in many vasculitides)
	CT sinuses in Wegener's granulomatosis
	Electromyography and nerve conduction studies
	Angiography (particularly Takayasu and polyarteritis nodosa)
	Tissue biopsy (renal, brain, peripheral nerve)

Management of mononeuritis multiplex is based on potent immunosuppression, often in the form of high-dose corticosteroids and cyclophosphamide, and the treatment of underlying infections such as hepatitis. This patient with foot drop will also require orthoses and physiotherapy to maximize physical function.

KEY POINTS

- Mononeuritis multiplex is commonly caused by diabetes or vasculitis.
- The vasculitides are classified according to size of the vessel involved.
- Mononeuritis multiplex due to vasculitis may require potent immunosuppression such as steroids and cyclophosphamide.

CASE 55: BACK PAIN AND THIRST IN AN ELDERLY MAN

History

A 72-year-old man is admitted to the emergency department with severe back pain. It started suddenly when he stepped awkwardly off his kitchen step, but he denies falling or direct injury to his spine. Apart from some vague discomfort in the back of his pelvis and hips for the last few months he has never had problems with his joints. On direct questioning, however, he does admit to some weight loss and feeling tired and 'washed out'. In addition he has been more thirsty than normal over the last few weeks, and he also complains of urinary frequency and nocturia.

Examination

This man is well but pale and in pain. He has marked bony tenderness over T11/12. His pelvis is not tender and his hips move freely. Neurological examination is normal. All other systems are also normal. Radiographs are shown in Figs 55.1 and 55.2.

INVESTIGATIONS		
		Normal range
Haemoglobin	7.9 g/dL	13.3–17.7 g/dL
Mean corpuscular volume (MCV)	88 fL	80–99 fL
White cell count	4.4×10^9/L	$3.9–10.6 \times 10^9$/L
Platelets	148×10^9/L	$150–440 \times 10^9$/L
ESR	104 mm/h	<10 mm/h
C-reactive protein	<5 mg/L	<5 mg/L
Urea	25.8 mmol/L	2.5–6.7 mmol/L
Creatinine	189 µmol/L	70–120 µmol/L
Corrected calcium	3.82 mmol/L	2.12–2.65 mmol/L

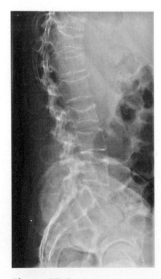

Figure 55.1

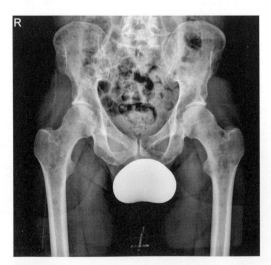

Figure 55.2

Questions

- Why was the X-ray performed and what does it show?
- What is the diagnosis?
- Can you link the blood test results to the clinical picture and radiology?
- How would you investigate and manage this patient?

ANSWER 55

This elderly man has presented with acute back pain and associated bony tenderness; an X-ray is therefore an appropriate investigation to attempt to identify a fracture, and to investigate the more longstanding pelvic/hip pain. The lateral spine X-ray demonstrates compression fractures at T11 and T12 which occurred after only minimal impact (suggesting skeletal fragility), and careful scrutiny of the whole spine reveals profound generalized osteopenia. In addition, the pelvic X-ray demonstrates well-defined lytic lesions throughout the pelvis and proximal femurs. The patient's blood tests demonstrate a marked normocytic anaemia (explaining his fatigue) and slightly reduced white cell and platelet counts, which therefore suggests a possible marrow disorder. His calcium is raised (resulting in thirst and nocturia) which may suggest a longstanding process affecting bone. Finally, the ESR is very elevated in the presence of a normal CRP, which might suggest a haematological process affecting erythrocyte sedimentation rather than a systemic inflammatory response. His renal impairment is pre-renal, which suggests an element of dehydration.

In summary, this elderly man has a combination of a normocytic anaemia, elevated calcium and a markedly elevated ESR plus widespread profound osteoporosis, lytic lesions and vertebral fractures. The most likely diagnosis is therefore multiple myeloma, a malignant proliferation of plasma cells (B-cells) which generates large quantities of antibody (immunoglobulin). The abnormal cell line threatens normal blood cell production which may lead to anaemia, leucopenia and/or thrombocytopenia; it induces enhanced osteoclast activity leading to osteoporosis, increased risk of fracture and hypercalcaemia, and the circulating light chains impair erythrocyte sedimentation, causing an isolated elevation of ESR and not the CRP. The main causes of renal impairment in myeloma are two-fold: not only does the elevation in serum calcium cause an osmotic diuresis and dehydration, but also the abnormal light chains may cause direct renal tubular damage.

A number of solid tumours (notably breast, lung, thyroid and kidney) may metastasize to bone; they may also produce an elevated calcium either through direct bony destruction or production of parathyroid hormone related protein (PTHrP). However, the overall picture in this case with evidence of marrow involvement suggests that myeloma is the most likely diagnosis.

The initial investigation of choice is immunoglobulins, serum electrophoresis and assessment of Bence–Jones protein (immunoglobulin light chains) in the urine. Patients with myeloma demonstrate a monoclonal gammopathy – classically IgG – with immune paresis (i.e. suppression of other immunoglobulins). The diagnostic test is bone marrow biopsy which reveals abnormal proliferation of plasma cells.

The immediate management of this patient would include:

- transfusion for anaemia
- rehydration for renal impairment
- rehydration and (if necessary bisphosphonates) for hypercalcaemia.

The patient should be referred to the haematology department for further treatment. Melphalan and prednisolone may induce a partial remission. High-dose chemotherapy with bone marrow transplantation may prolong survival but is not routinely offered to those over the age of 55 years as the associated mortality rate of the therapy is up to 40 per cent.

KEY POINTS

- The combination of bone pain and elevated ESR and calcium is suggestive of multiple myeloma.
- Myeloma is an important cause of osteoporosis.
- Screening tests for myeloma are immunoglobulins, serum electrophoresis and Bence–Jones protein in the urine.
- Myeloma is diagnosed by bone marrow biopsy.

CASE 56: ACUTE BACK PAIN

History

A 58-year-old woman presents to the emergency department with acute back pain. She stumbled off a step and, although she denies falling or receiving direct trauma to the spine, she developed acute and severe mid-thoracic pain immediately afterwards. Her past medical history is unremarkable. She admits to drinking up to 30 units of alcohol a week and smokes 30 cigarettes per day.

Examination

This woman is thin and in considerable pain. The pain is central with no radiation. There are no peripheral stigmata of systemic disease and cardiovascular, respiratory, abdominal and neurological examinations are normal. She has a marked kyphosis and has point tenderness over several thoracic vertebrae. A radiograph is shown in Fig. 56.1.

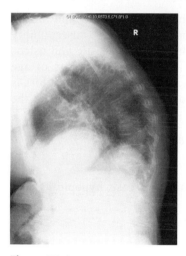

Figure 56.1

Questions

- What is the diagnosis?
- What risk factors for this disorder does she already have, and what other factors should be specifically sought in the history?
- How would you investigate and manage this patient?

ANSWER 56

Although a number of medical and surgical conditions can give rise to pain radiating to the back, this patient's pain is reproducible by pressure on the vertebral bodies, suggesting a bony origin for her symptoms, and the X-ray reveals several so-called wedge fractures of the vertebral bodies at the sites of maximal tenderness. Given the injury was sustained following minimal and indirect impact, one must consider skeletal fragility in this case.

Skeletal fragility may be localized due to a malignant deposit giving rise to a pathological fracture (and given her smoking history this might be a possibility), but reassuringly there is no radiological evidence of a lytic destructive lesion around the fractures. Nonetheless it would be appropriate to look for a history of cough or haemoptysis and to enquire about recent weight loss or whether she has always been slim. If there were any suggestive symptoms in her history you should consider performing a chest X-ray. Otherwise (and since there is no radiological evidence of a bony malignancy) the most likely explanation of fracture in this case is widespread skeletal fragility due to osteoporosis.

Osteoporosis is a systemic skeletal disease characterized by low bone mass and micro-architectural deterioration of bone tissue with increase in bone fragility and susceptibility to fracture. Bone mass or mineral density relies on a balance of osteoblastic and osteoclastic activity. Overall it peaks in adulthood and then declines from 35 years of age onwards, accelerating in women following the menopause. Postmenopausal bone loss is the most common cause of osteoporosis, but secondary osteoporosis may occur in the context of a number of medical conditions:

- postmenopausal oestrogen deficiency (most common cause)
- amenorrhoea
- iatrogenic (corticosteroid therapy)
- endocrine (hyperparathyroidism, hyperthyroidism, Cushing's disease, hypopituitarism, hypogonadism)
- malabsorption (e.g. coeliac disease)
- osteomalacia
- multiple myeloma
- inflammatory arthropathy (probably due to elevated IL-1 and/or TNF-α).

This patient has a number of risk factors for osteoporosis in the form of a low body mass index (BMI) and a history of smoking and excess alcohol. The major risk factors that should be specifically sought in the history of a patient with suspected osteoporosis are:

- maternal family history of hip fracture
- oestrogen deficiency (e.g. premature menopause, prolonged secondary amenorrhoea)
- corticosteroid therapy with a prednisolone dose >7.5 mg/day for over 6 months
- low BMI (<19 kg/m^2), due to a combination of reduced oestrogen levels and reduction in impact loading
- smoking and excess alcohol
- anorexia nervosa
- prolonged immobilization.

Osteoporosis is diagnosed and severity determined using a dual-energy X-ray absorptiometry or DEXA scan. This compares bone mineral density (BMD) at the lumbar spine and proximal femur with that of the young normal mean – the *T* score:

- Normal – BMD <1 standard deviation (SD) below young normal mean
- osteopenia – BMD 1–2.5 SDs below young normal mean

- osteoporosis – BMD >2.5 SDs below young normal mean
- severe osteoporosis – as above plus previous fragility fracture.

The present patient should have a DEXA scan and, like any other patient with confirmed osteoporosis, should undergo screening investigations for the secondary causes of low bone mass. Thyroid function tests, a myeloma screen, vitamin D level, bone and hormonal profile would be considered essential.

The pain due to acute vertebral collapse can be severe and may require opiates; if persistent, vertebroplasty (the injection of bone cement directly into the fractured vertebral body) may prove beneficial. Osteoporosis treatment is aimed at reducing falls and skeletal fragility. Lifestyle modifications such as weight-bearing exercise, smoking cessation and alcohol reduction are all critical.

Pharmacological treatment in the form of calcium supplementation and bisphosphonates to reduce osteoclast activity is effective but compliance is typically poor. All patients receiving corticosteroids should have bone protection as, for a given BMD, osteoporosis caused by steroids has the highest rate of fractures. Alternatives to bisphosphonate therapy for the treatment of osteoporosis include selective oestrogen receptor modulators (SERMs, e.g. raloxifene), strontium and teriparatide (a synthetic PTH). Hormone replacement therapy (HRT) may be beneficial in primary prevention of osteoporosis but is not of proven benefit in established disease.

 KEY POINTS

- Osteoporosis is a condition of low bone mineral density leading to skeletal fragility.
- The most common cause is postmenopausal oestrogen deficiency.
- Steroid-induced osteoporosis is a significant problem in medical practice. Never forget bone protection in patients receiving corticosteroids!

CASE 57: PAINFUL BONES AND A WADDLING GAIT

History

A 45-year-old Asian woman is referred to the rheumatology department with generalized bone pain and difficulty walking. She denies localized joint pain but 'hurts all over', and she finds it hard to get out of a chair or climb the stairs and walks with a waddling gait. Her symptoms have been getting progressively worse for around a year. She is otherwise well.

Examination

This woman has no peripheral stigmata of inflammatory disease and has bone rather than joint tenderness. She has mild proximal weakness. The remainder of the examination is normal.

INVESTIGATIONS		
		Normal range
ESR	4 mm/h	<10 mm/h
CRP	<5 mg/L	<5 mg/L
Creatine kinase	54 iU/L	25–195 iU/L
Ca	2.04 mmol/L	2.12–2.65 mmol/L
Phosphate	0.7 mmol/L	0.8–1.45 mmol/L
Alkaline phosphatase	456 iU/L	30–300 iU/L
25-hydroxyvitamin D	8.1 nmol/L	12.5–350 nmol/L
Parathyroid hormone	7.3 pmol/L	1.0–6.1 pmol/L

Questions

- What is the diagnosis?
- What are the potential risk factors in this case?
- What is the differential diagnosis of bone pain and weakness?
- How would you manage this patient?

ANSWER 57

This patient has a combination of bone pain and proximal myopathy. The normal CK suggests that it is not a primary muscle disorder and the biochemical picture of low vitamin D and high PTH suggests vitamin D deficiency. The diagnosis is osteomalacia, a condition of poor mineralization of bone and excessive osteoid. The symptoms of osteomalacia can be very vague and the condition must be specifically considered to avoid missing the diagnosis.

! Features of osteomalacia and rickets	
Bone pain/tenderness	Particularly in ribs (may wake patient when turning during sleep)
Proximal myopathy	Power may also be limited by bone pain
Paraesthesiae or tetany	Due to hypocalcaemia
Radiology	Looser zone in osteomalacia (translucent ribbon of failed mineralization)
Biochemistry	Low vitamin D
	Low or normal calcium and phosphate
	High alkaline phosphatase and parathyroid hormone

! Features of rickets alone	
Deformity	Craniotabes of the skull (soft and compressible skull)
	Frontal and parietal bossing
	Enlarged epiphyses
	Rickety rosary of osteochondral junctions
	Harrison's sulcus in the rib cage
	Bowed or knock-knees

The most common cause of vitamin D deficiency is lack of sun exposure (UV radiation on skin is necessary for its production from 7-dehydroxycholesterol precursor in the skin) which is common in those who cover up due to religious reasons and those living in institutions, including the elderly. Possible risk factors for osteomalacia in this case are religious covering of the skin plus a high intake of chapati – the flour used contains phytanic acid which binds calcium and may therefore increase vitamin D requirements. The causes of osteomalacia are listed below.

! Causes of osteomalacia
• Low vitamin D: lack of sun exposure, poor oral intake
• Malabsorption: coeliac disease, gastrectomy, pancreatic insufficiency
• Renal disease: renal osteodystrophy, hypophosphataemic renal disease, Fanconi syndrome, renal tubular acidosis
• Drugs: anticonvulsants (phenytoin and carbamazepine)

The differential diagnosis of osteomalacia is extensive and includes:

- fibromyalgia
- osteoporosis
- polymyalgia rheumatica
- polymyositis
- rheumatoid arthritis
- multiple myeloma
- metastatic bone disease.

The lack of inflammatory response and a normal CK is therefore very reassuring in the assessment of a patient with possible osteomalacia.

Management of osteomalacia focuses on patient education. Only minimal sun exposure (15 minutes of sunshine to face and hands/arms) is required to maintain vitamin D levels, although those with darker skin will require longer exposure. Oily fish and certain supplemented cereals should be included in the diet wherever possible, but frank vitamin D deficiency is treated with supplementation. Mild deficiency is treated with 800 iu vitamin D daily, but more severe deficiency requires a high-dose oral bolus followed by standard daily doses. All patients with vitamin D supplementation should also receive additional calcium.

 KEY POINTS

- Osteomalacia is due to vitamin D deficiency.
- The symptoms may be very non-specific.
- Osteomalacia is common in certain ethnic groups and those living in institutions.

CASE 58: HIP PAIN AND ABNORMAL BLOOD TESTS

History
A 78-year-old man is referred to the rheumatology department by his general practitioner. He has been complaining of hip pain for some months. His GP suspected osteoarthritis and arranged for some screening bloods and a pelvic X-ray (Fig. 58.1). The pain has settled somewhat with analgesia but his X-ray was abnormal and precipitated the referral for advice on diagnosis and management.

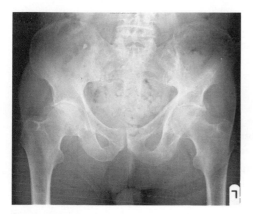

Figure 58.1

INVESTIGATIONS		
		Normal range
ESR	<10 mm/h	<10 mm/h
CRP	<5 mg/l	<5 mg/L
Urea	6.4 mmol/L	2.5–6.7 mmol/L
Creatinine	72 µmol/L	70–120 µmol/L
Bilirubin	12 µmol/L	3–17 µmol/L
Alanine aminotransferase	32 iU/L	5–35 iU/L
Alkaline phosphatase	976 iU/L	30–300 iU/L
Calcium	2.45 mmol/L	2.12–2.65 mmol/L

Questions
- What is the likely diagnosis?
- What are the potential complications?
- How would you manage this patient?

ANSWER 58

This elderly man has a very abnormal pelvic X-ray with evidence of loss of trabeculae, abnormally thickened bone and sclerosis. In combination with his history of bone pain and an elevated alkaline phosphatase (ALP), the most likely diagnosis is Paget's disease.

Paget's disease is a condition of disordered bone remodelling with increased osteoclast and osteoblast activity. Indeed, it is the accelerated osteoblast activity that gives rise to the elevated ALP. Although most commonly asymptomatic, the bone architecture in Paget's is mosaic-like and mechanically weaker than normal bone; as a result, bone deformities (e.g. tibial bowing) or spontaneous fractures may result. Paget's bone is also hypervascular and may feel warm to palpation. The majority of Paget's (80 per cent) is polyostotic, affecting several bones simultaneously; when the disease is isolated to a single site, the tibia and iliac bones are the most commonly affected areas.

! Complications of Paget's disease	
Skeletal	Bone pain
	Deformity (bowing, skull enlargement)
	Fracture
Neurological (compression syndromes)	Deafness
	Spinal or cranial nerve entrapment
	Spinal stenosis
Cardiovascular	Hyperthermia and warmth of affected area
	High-output congestive cardiac failure
	Carotid steal syndrome (to Pagetic skull)
Malignant change	Osteogenic sarcoma
Metabolic	Hypercalcaemia (in the presence of fracture or immobility)

The diagnosis of Paget's disease is the combination of radiological and biochemical abnormalities. Plain X-rays reveal mixtures of sclerotic and lytic lesions and significant trabecular thickening. 'Osteoporosis circumscripta' refers to extensive lytic disease affecting the skull. Full-body scintigraphy may be used to determine the extent of disease as affected areas show marked increased uptake.

In practical terms, the main indication to treat Paget's disease is pain – as in this case – although bone deformity or compression syndromes (or risk thereof) would also prompt therapy. The treatment of choice is a bisphosphonate to diminish osteoclast activity, interrupting the vicious cycle of chaotic bone remodelling. Intravenous zolendronate is highly effective in this regard and serum ALP and type 1 procollagen (P1NP) levels are sensitive markers of bone formation and are suppressed during successful treatment. Patients should be regularly reviewed for changes in symptoms or elevation of these biochemical markers: either would be an indication for re-treatment.

 KEY POINTS

- Paget's disease may be diagnosed incidentally on X-ray.
- Treatment is for bone pain or other complications.
- The intravenous bisphosphonate zolendronate is the treatment of choice.

CASE 59: KNEE PAIN IN AN ATHLETE

History

A 36-year-old recreational runner presents with anterior knee pain. She has recently increased training in preparation for a marathon and runs exclusively on roads. A few weeks prior to presentation she developed crescendo knee pain while running which did not resolve when she stopped. The pain is now also present at rest. She is otherwise well with no previous injuries but did experience 8 months of secondary amenorrhoea due to overtraining in her early twenties. Since then her periods have been normal. She does not smoke or drink and is on no regular medication although she has been taking paracetamol for the pain.

Examination

This patient has a normal gait but is unable to hop on the affected side because of the pain. There is an area of focal bony tenderness in the medial proximal tibia. Examination of her knee and other joints is normal.

Questions

- What is the likely diagnosis?
- What is the investigation of choice?
- What is the differential diagnosis of anterior knee pain?
- How would you manage this patient?

ANSWER 59

The most likely diagnosis is a stress fracture of the proximal tibia. Stress fractures are overuse injuries and occur when periosteal resorption exceeds bone formation. They are commonly seen in two main patient groups: soldiers may suffer so-called march fractures in the metatarsals, while athletes may develop them in different sites according to their sporting activity. Although the knee is a common site in runners due to excess mechanical loading, stress fractures may also result in non-weight-bearing sites due to repetitive and excessive traction (e.g. rib fractures in rowers due to traction from serratus anterior). The classic symptom – as in this case – is of pain that occurs throughout running and crucially persists with rest; this is in contrast to shin splints, a traction injury to the tibial periosteum in which the pain diminishes somewhat with continued activity, only to return again after the patient has stopped running.

The investigation of choice is CT or MRI as radiographs are frequently normal.

The differential diagnosis of anterior knee pain is extensive and includes:

- patellar maltracking and malalignment
- chondromalacia patellae (a degenerative condition of patellar cartilage)
- patellar tendinopathy
- pre- or infrapatellar bursitis
- meniscal damage
- tight iliotibial band
- referred pain from the hip or lumbosacral spine.

The management of stress fractures is rest until the pain has completely settled and focal tenderness has resolved. For those with severe stress fractures in the lower limb, an air-cast boot can offer support and assist in a gradual resumption of weight-bearing. The crucial feature of rehabilitation is a graded return to sport to prevent progression or recurrence. Patients with stress fractures should also undergo a thorough physiotherapy assessment to identify and treat any predisposing biomechanical factors. In addition this patient already has a history of overtraining and so one should remain alert for the development of the 'female athlete triad' of disordered eating, amenorrhoea and osteoporosis. Many physicians would screen any stress fracture patient with a clinical assessment of osteoporosis risk followed by a DEXA scan and assessment of serological bone profile (calcium, alkaline phosphatase and vitamin D status).

 KEY POINTS

- Stress fractures are overuse injuries and common in athletes.
- Patients with stress fractures should be assessed for osteoporosis.
- Consider the female athlete triad in any woman with a stress fracture.

CASE 60: PAINFUL HANDS AND A RASH

History

A 38-year-old man visits his general practitioner with a 2-month history of painful hands. It developed insidiously over a few weeks and affects primarily the distal and proximal interphalangeal joints in his hands, the whole of his third toe on the right foot and his right heel. The pain, stiffness and swelling are most marked in the morning but improve with exercise and ibuprofen. His past medical history is unremarkable. Systemic enquiry reveals a longstanding rash which affects his forearms and umbilicus for which he uses emollients.

Examination

There are plaques of scaly skin affecting his forearms, scalp and umbilicus. His nails are dystrophic with pitting and ridging and there is soft-tissue swelling and synovitis affecting the distal and proximal interphalangeal joints. He has a 'sausage toe' on the right foot. His right Achilles tendon is swollen and tender in its distal third, with pain on palpation of the insertion into the calcaneum.

INVESTIGATIONS		
		Normal range
Rheumatoid factor (RF)	Negative	
Anti-citrullinated protein antibody (ACPA)	Negative	
ESR	8	<10 mm/h
CRP	<5 mg/L	<5 mg/L

Questions

- What is the differential diagnosis of arthropathy and a rash?
- Which is the most likely here?
- Are the normal inflammatory markers unusual?
- What treatment is available?

ANSWER 60

Arthropathy and rash is a common combination in rheumatology, so a detailed system enquiry is crucial. Not only will the systems review highlight the associated rash which may not be immediately apparent, but it may also reveal other features (e.g. ocular or gastrointestinal involvement) of a unifying diagnosis.

The most likely differential diagnosis for rash and arthropathy is psoriatic arthritis, systemic lupus erythematosus, vasculitis, sarcoidosis and enteric arthropathy. Other possibilities include infections such as gonococcal arthritis, Lyme disease, rheumatic fever or infective endocarditis. By far the most likely unifying diagnosis in this case is psoriatic arthritis as the rash, nail and joint involvement are characteristic. The seronegativity (i.e. RF and ACPA negative) is also very supportive.

Psoriatic arthritis is a common inflammatory arthropathy that affects up to 15 per cent of those with psoriasis. It has a number of characteristic presentations and clinical features that can help to differentiate between true psoriatic arthropathy and those with psoriasis and another inflammatory arthropathy such as rheumatoid arthritis. Although the following are the 'classic' psoriatic presentations, patients may have several overlapping features from different categories.

! **Clinical features of psoriatic arthropathy**

- Dactylitis or 'sausage' digit and (insertional) tendinopathy
- Distal polyarticular disease (predominantly involving distal and proximal interphalangeal joints)
- Proximal polyarticular disease (predominantly involving metacarpophalangeal and proximal interphalangeal joints, very similar to rheumatoid)
- Sacroiliitis and/or spondyloarthropathy
- Oligoarthritis (particularly hips and knees)
- Arthritis mutilans with marked osteolysis and telescoping of the digits

---

The rash may be very mild, overlooked and under-reported, so clinical examination of a patient with possible psoriatic arthritis should include careful scrutiny of the typically affected sites such as hairline or natal cleft. Indeed, nail changes may be the only clinical evidence of psoriasis and are an invaluable adjunct to diagnosis; changes include pitting, ridging and onycholysis.

Diagnosis rests on a typical history and clinical examination; there is no diagnostic test and often the acute phase is not as marked as in other inflammatory joint diseases – as in this case. Radiology is unhelpful early on: the periarticular osteopenia of rheumatoid is characteristically absent and the classic osteolysis leading to 'pencil-in-cup' deformities is a late feature. Tendinopathy, enthesopathy, plantar fasciitis, sacroiliitis and spondylo-arthropathy may be evident on MRI.

Treatment is similar to that for rheumatoid arthritis. Disease-modifying agents such as methotrexate and leflunomide are used first-line (while hydroxychloroquine tends to be avoided as it may exacerbate skin disease). For patients with active disease despite an adequate trial of DMARDs TNF-α blockade is very beneficial, for both skin and joints. Since this patient also has disease affecting the Achilles tendon, a prompt ultrasound scan to determine severity of inflammation and tendon integrity would be important. Steroid injections are relatively contraindicated in weight-bearing tendons as the risk of rupture is profound, so emergency treatment for an at-risk tendon is immobilization in an air-cast boot.

KEY POINTS

- Rash and arthropathy are common presenting complaints.
- The most common differential is psoriatic arthritis.
- Nail disease is very helpful in differentiating psoriatic arthritis from other forms of inflammatory arthropathy.
- Psoriatic arthritis has a number of clinical patterns. Distal small-joint disease is the most common.

CASE 61: HYPERMOBILITY AND A PNEUMOTHORAX

History

A 19-year-old man is referred by the chest team following admission with a spontaneous pneumothorax. He has made a full recovery but during his admission it was noted that he has hypermobile joints, long digits and possible skin laxity.

Examination

This young man is tall, with disproportionately long limbs and long fingers. He has a pectus excavatum and a mild scoliosis. His palate is high-arching and there is dental overcrowding. His skin, including a scar from a minor injury, appears normal.

Questions

- How is hypermobility formally assessed?
- What diagnosis does the patient's appearance and pneumothorax suggest?
- What is the feared complication?
- Which related condition is associated with hypermobility, skin laxity and abnormal scar formation?

ANSWER 61

Hypermobility (or hyperextensibility) can be assessed using Beighton's criteria. If 4 out of 9 points are scored on the following criteria, the patient is regarded as having joint laxity:

- knee extension more than 10 degrees past 180 degreees (2 points)
- extension of the elbow 10 degrees past 180 degrees (2 points)
- extension of the thumb to touch the anterior forearm (2 points)
- extension of the fifth finger backward to 90 degrees (2 points)
- trunk flexion with palms flat on the floor (1 point).

A degree of joint laxity is not uncommon in the normal population but it may occur as part of a wider spectrum of the heritable collagen diseases. The most common of these are Marfan and Ehlers–Danlos syndromes. This patient's phenotype and history of spontaneous pneumothorax, however, are characteristic of Marfan syndrome.

Marfan syndrome is due to a defect in the fibrillin gene, leading to an abnormal elastin substructure. It results in abnormalities in a number of systems (see below). Although it is an autosomal dominant condition, up to 25 per cent of cases are due to a spontaneous mutation.

! Clinical features of Marfan syndrome	
Skeletal	Tall and thin
	Disproportionally long legs
	Arachnodactyly (spider fingers)
	Pectus carinatum or excavatum
	Loss of thoracic kyphosis
	Scoliosis
	High-arched palate with dental overcrowding
Ocular	Ectopialentis (upward dislocation of the lens)
Cardiovascular	Aortic dilatation and dissection
	Mitral valve prolapse
Pulmonary	Spontaneous pneumothorax
	Apical blebs
Cutaneous	Incisional hernia
	Stretch marks (in absence of weight change or pregnancy)
Radiological	Dural ectasia (enlargement of dural sac)

The most feared complication is of aortic dissection, so all patients with Marfan syndrome should have annual screening by echocardiography and early consideration of elective repair. Patients with mitral valve prolapse are at risk of endocarditis.

The other main differential in this case, Ehlers–Danlos syndrome, is a collagen defect leading to joint laxity and skin fragility/hyperextensibility. These patients have velvety-feeling skin with poor healing characteristics leading to gaping ('fish-mouth') scars and easy bruising. The feared complication in this patient group is aneurysm formation and arterial rupture due to elastic tissue laxity.

KEY POINTS

- Joint hypermobility is common in the normal population, particularly young girls.
- Hypermobility is assessed using Beighton's criteria.
- Marfan syndrome is characterized by hypermobility and skeletal disproportion.

CASE 62: PINS AND NEEDLES IN A YOUNG WOMAN

History

A 28-year-old woman with a 10-year history of rheumatoid arthritis is reviewed in clinic. She is 30 weeks' gestation in her first pregnancy and stopped all her disease-modifying agents prior to conception. Her arthritis has remained quiescent, but over the last few weeks she has become troubled by pins and needles over the lateral half of her right hand. The symptoms are particularly prominent at night and settle when she shakes her hand. There is no early morning stiffness and her grip strength is unaffected, but she is finding her work as a piano teacher increasingly difficult.

INVESTIGATIONS		
		Normal range
Haemoglobin	14.9 g/dL	13.3–17.7 g/dL
White cell count	7.4×10^9/L	$3.9–10.6 \times 10^9$/L
Platelets	323×10^9/L	$150–440 \times 10^9$/L
ESR	8 mm/h	<10 mm/h
CRP	3 mg/L	<5 mg/L

Questions

- What is the diagnosis?
- Identify two risk factors for this in the patient's history.
- What would you look for on examination?
- How would you investigate and manage the patient?

ANSWER 62

This is a very good description of carpal tunnel syndrome. Carpal tunnel syndrome is the most common entrapment neuropathy, in which the median nerve becomes compressed beneath the flexor retinaculum on its route to the hand. The classic symptoms are of tingling in the sensory distribution of the median nerve (i.e. the lateral three and a half digits); loss of thumb abduction is a late feature. Symptoms are often worse at night (when the hand might be quite painful) and in certain postures such as holding a newspaper or driving.

The majority of cases are idiopathic, but pregnancy and rheumatoid arthritis are very common precipitating causes – as in this case. Other common conditions to consider are acromegaly, hypothyroidism and diabetes. Carpal tunnel syndrome is also more common in those whose occupation risks mechanical overuse, such as piano players!

Examination should start with general 'end of the bed' observation for signs of associated conditions. On inspection of the hands there may be wasting of the thenar eminence. Sensory change is detectable over the palmar aspects of the first three and a half digits and there may be weakness of abduction, flexion and opposition of the thumb. Tinel's sign occurs when tapping the palmar aspect of the affected wrist produces paraesthesia distally; Phalen's sign is positive when maximal flexion of the affected wrist provokes or exacerbates the symptoms. Both these tests have limited sensitivity and specificity but may lend weight to the diagnosis. Although she denies early-morning stiffness and has a normal inflammatory response, a clinical assessment of her RA disease activity is crucial to determine whether synovitis is contributing to the entrapment syndrome. The gold standard investigation is a nerve conduction study which will demonstrate (and quantify) reduction in conduction velocity through the carpal tunnel.

The majority of patients will respond well to conservative management, such as avoidance of provoking activities and wrist splints (particularly at night). This approach would be entirely suitable in this case as her symptoms may settle post-partum. If these measures fail, corticosteroid injection into the carpal tunnel can be very effective in up to 80 per cent of patients. Surgical decompression should be reserved for those with persistent disabling symptoms or motor loss.

 KEY POINTS

- Carpal tunnel syndrome is an entrapment neuropathy of the median nerve.
- It characteristically produces paraesthesia in the lateral three and a half digits.
- The diagnostic test is nerve conduction studies.
- Treatment may be conservative, steroid injection or surgical decompression.

CASE 63: JOINT PAINS, SKIN CHANGES AND MUSCLE WEAKNESS

History

A 44-year-old woman presents to the rheumatology department with a constellation of symptoms. She was well until 8 months ago when she developed Raynaud's phenomenon and joint pains. The latter responded to a non-steroidal anti-inflammatory drug (NSAID), so she 'got on with normal life'. Over the last few months she has noticed the skin over her fingers becoming tighter. In recent weeks she has developed muscle weakness such that she finds it difficult to climb stairs or get out of a chair unaided.

Examination

There is some skin tethering over the fingers, with reduction in the finger pulps. Although her joints are painful there is no objective evidence of synovitis. Proximal muscle power is reduced to 3/5. Respiratory examination reveals fine inspiratory crackles bibasally, but the remainder of her examination is normal. The general practitioner who referred her performed an 'autoimmune screen'.

INVESTIGATIONS	
ANA	Positive
Anti-dsDNA	Negative
Anti-Ro	Negative
Anti-La	Negative
Anti-Sm	Negative
Anti-U1-RNP	Positive
Polyclonal hypergammaglobulinaemia	

Questions

- What is the likely diagnosis?
- What further investigations might you initiate?
- How would you manage this patient?

ANSWER 63

This female patient has presented with a combination of features seen in RA, SLE, myositis and scleroderma in the presence of anti-U1-RNP antibodies. The most likely diagnosis is, therefore, mixed connective tissue disease (MCTD). Whether MCTD remains a truly distinct clinical entity is somewhat controversial and many patients may eventually develop sufficient features to fulfil established diagnostic criteria of a particular autoimmune disease. The case presented here highlights the most common presenting features for MCTD:

- joint symptoms
- Raynaud's phenomenon
- sclerodactyly
- proximal myopathy.

Other frequent problems include oesophageal dysmotility, serositis and lymphadenopathy.

Although respiratory involvement is common in MCTD, it is often asymptomatic. This patient has fine bibasal crackles, which is suggestive of interstitial lung disease. She will need a chest X-ray and possibly a high-resolution CT scan to identify interstitial changes, as well as lung function studies to quantify any restrictive defect or reduced gas transfer (diffusion capacity).

Management of MCTD involves directing therapy at specific abnormalities. The treatment for each clinical feature in the combination is identical to that for a given presentation in isolation; for example, vasodilators for Raynaud's phenomenon, hydroxychloroquine for arthralgia, and corticosteroids for myositis. Over time, the inflammatory component and severity of MCTD manifestations generally diminish. Pulmonary hypertension is the leading cause of disease-associated death.

 KEY POINTS

- Mixed connective tissue disease is characterized by the presence of anti-U1-RNP antibodies.
- Most common features of this mixed clinical picture are arthralgia, Raynaud's phenomenon, sclerodactyly and proximal myopathy.
- Pulmonary hypertension is the most feared complication.

CASE 64: AN ACUTELY PAINFUL KNEE

History

A 56-year-old man presents to the emergency department with a 2-day history of an acutely painful, swollen and hot knee. He is otherwise well but felt feverish on the morning of his admission. There is no history of trauma and the systems enquiry is unremarkable. Past medical history includes left ventricular failure, hypertension and renal impairment. Current medications are aspirin, furosemide and ramipril. He lives alone, smokes 15 cigarettes per day and drinks 30 units of alcohol per week.

Examination

This man is uncomfortable but well. His temperature is 37.1°C, pulse 110/min and blood pressure 145/83 mmHg. General examination is unremarkable, but his right knee is warm with a tense effusion. Both passive and active movement are restricted by pain, and weight-bearing is uncomfortable. Other joints are normal.

INVESTIGATIONS		
		Normal range
Haemoglobin	15.9 g/dL	13.3–17.7 g/dL
White cell count	11.2 × 10⁹/L	3.9–10.6 × 10⁹/L
Platelets	523 × 10⁹/L	150–440 × 10⁹/L
ESR	24 mm/h	<10 mm/h
CRP	94 mg/L	<5 mg/L
Urea	19.8 mmol/L	2.5–6.7 mmol/l
Creatinine	152 µmol/L	70–120 µmol/L
Urate	278 µmol/L	240–400 µmol/L

Questions

• What are the top differential diagnoses to consider and which is most likely?
• What is the investigation of choice?

ANSWER 64

In any patient presenting with an acutely painful and swollen joint, the most important diagnoses to consider are septic arthritis and crystal arthropathy. Crystal arthropathy such as gout is more common than septic arthritis; and since this patient is well with no discernible risk factors for sepsis, it is the most likely diagnosis here. The investigation of choice is a prompt aspiration of the joint with assessment of the synovial fluid for crystals or bacteria (and if the latter are detected, culture to determine the causative organism and its sensitivity to antibiotics).

Crystal arthropathy is caused by either uric acid (gout) or pyrophosphate (pseudo-gout) crystals precipitating out into the synovial fluid, generating a brisk inflammatory response. The classic clinical picture is discrete attacks of monoarticular inflammation – often initially the metatarsophalangeal joint – followed by asymptomatic periods; in more severe, longstanding cases, the disease can become polyarticular. Risk factors for gout are under-excretion or over-production of urate, which is a product of DNA break-down and present in large amounts in certain foods and alcohol. Urate crystals may also deposit in the skin, causing painful discrete lumps known as tophi, or in the renal tract, causing urate nephropathy or lithiasis.

! Causes of over-production and under-excretion of urate	
Over-production	*Under-excretion*
Excess alcohol	Excess alcohol
High consumption of meat and shellfish	Renal impairment
Chemotherapy	Loop diuretics
Haematological malignancy	Low-dose aspirin
Psoriasis	

Investigations will reveal an elevated acute-phase response, often with a neutrophilia and thrombocytosis due to the inflammatory response (although this can lead to diagnostic confusion with septic arthritis). The urate level may be normal during an acute attack and is therefore relatively unhelpful. Microscopy of the synovial fluid will reveal needle-shaped crystals that are negatively birefringent on polarized microscopy in cases of gout, and positively birefringent brick-shaped crystals in pyrophosphate disease. It is worth bearing in mind that crystals can occur as innocent bystanders in infection; so unless the diagnosis is clear-cut, it is worth sending a synovial fluid sample for culture. In chronic disease, X-rays may reveal the classic punched-out erosions with sclerotic margins. Osteopenia is characteristically absent. Pyrophosphate arthropathy may be associated with radiological evidence of chondrocalcinosis.

Treatment of an acute attack includes anti-inflammatories such as non-steroidal anti-inflammatories (NSAIDs), colchicine or steroids, depending on the patient's comorbidities. In this case, for example, the renal impairment is a relative contraindication for NSAIDs, so low-dose colchicine or a short course of oral prednisolone might be appropriate. Injection of the affected joint with corticosteroid and local anaesthetic will also offer immediate and effective relief and should be offered to all patients in whom there is no evidence of septic disease. In cases of gout, patients should be given lifestyle advice which can have a huge effect on urate levels (e.g. reducing alcohol and meat intake) and, where possible, offending medications should be stopped or switched to alternatives with no impact on urate handling. Long-term treatment with urate-lowering therapy such as allopurinol should be commenced if the patient experiences recurrent attacks, but its commencement can precipitate another gout attack and should be started only when an acute attack is over and under anti-inflammatory cover. There is no long-term prophy-laxis for pyrophosphate disease.

KEY POINTS

- Crystal arthropathy is a common cause of an acutely painful joint (but always consider and rule out septic arthritis).
- Gout may be precipitated by diuretics, renal impairment and aspirin use, so is a common clinical problem in general medicine.
- Diagnosis is based on identification of urate crystals in synovial fluid; serum levels may be normal.
- Acute treatment relies on NSAIDS, colchicine or steroids.
- Lifestyle modification may prevent further attacks. If not, commence allopurinol under anti-inflammatory cover.

CASE 65: RECURRENT ABDOMINAL PAIN AND FEVERS

History

A 16-year-old Turkish boy is seen in the emergency department with abdominal pain and fever. His right knee is also exquisitely tender and slightly swollen. He has suffered recurrent attacks with a similar presentation since childhood, although normally they are more severe and also include pleurisy. He has been told that 'it runs in the family'. The attacks resolve spontaneously and in between times he is entirely well.

Examination

This adolescent is very uncomfortable, with a temperature of 38.8°C. His pulse rate is 110/min, blood pressure 115/63 mmHg. He has marked abdominal tenderness with rebound and guarding; his bowel sounds are reduced. There is a mild and cool effusion of his right knee, which is extremely tender. The rest of his examination is normal.

Questions

- What diagnosis might explain recurrent abdominal pain, pleurisy and fever?
- How would you investigate this patient?
- What is the feared complication of the underlying diagnosis?
- How would you treat this patient?

ANSWER 65

The admitting senior house officer decided to refer this adolescent to the surgical team as an acute abdomen. Although the SHO made the right decision to admit under the surgical team, it is worth keeping an open mind to the diagnosis in view of its recurrent nature and family history. The combination of recurrent serositis (peritonitis and pleuritis), fever and eastern Mediterranean origin raises the possibility of familial Mediterranean fever (FMF) as the underlying diagnosis.

FMF is an autosomal recessively inherited periodic syndrome characterized by stereo-typed attacks of fever and inflammatory features which last up to 4 days and then remit spontaneously. The most common manifestations are:

- fever
- peritonitis
- arthritis
- pleuritis
- rash (erysipelas-like).

The arthritis is classically monoarticular and symptoms often outweigh the signs, with extreme tenderness despite only mild effusions and a marked absence of increased temperature.

This patient should still be investigated for acute abdomen with blood tests including inflammatory markers, amylase and lactate and imaging in the form of an abdominal and erect chest X-ray. Patients in whom one suspects FMF should be referred to a specialist centre for genetic testing.

One of the feared complications of FMF is the development of amyloidosis. Amyloidosis is a multisystem disease caused by the deposition of insoluble protein in the extracellular matrix: renal, cardiac and hepatic tissues are commonly affected. Primary amyloid (AL) is formed from deposition of immunoglobulin light chains and occurs in isolation or in the context of myeloma. Secondary or reactive amyloid (AA) is caused by the deposition of amyloid A rather than light chains and may complicate any chronic infective, malignant or inflammatory process such as FMF.

Colchicine is the treatment of choice. It is not only very effective at diminishing the attacks of serositis in FMF, but has also been shown to reduce the development of renal amyloidosis in these patients by up to two-thirds.

 KEY POINTS

- Consider a periodic syndrome in anyone presenting with recurrent serositis and fever.
- The arthritis in FMF often generates a greater level of pain than one would expect from the clinical signs.

CASE 66: PAINFUL HANDS AND ORAL ULCERS

History

A 27-year-old Afro-Caribbean woman presents to the rheumatology clinic with a long history of painful hands and oral ulcers. She feels she 'hasn't been well' for many years with various problems including chest pains, occasional rashes and hair loss. She recently visited her family in Jamaica and felt much worse, with a resurgence of all of her symptoms, particularly the rash. She is currently experiencing an attack of her typical central chest pain which is sharp and relieved by sitting forward.

Examination

This young woman is uncomfortable and slightly short of breath. Pulse is 115/min sinus rhythm, blood pressure 95/62 mmHg, and oxygen saturation 98 per cent on room air. Her jugular venous pressure (JVP) is elevated at 2 cm and her heart sounds are quiet with no added sounds. Chest examination reveals stony dull bases with reduced vocal resonance and diminished breath sounds.

INVESTIGATIONS		
		Normal range
Haemoglobin	13.2 g/dL	13.3–17.7 g/dL
White cell count	2.6×10^9/L	3.9–10.6×10^9/L
Platelets	98×10^9/L	150–440×10^9/L
ESR	84 mm/h	<10 mm/h
CRP	20 mg/L	<5 mg/L
ANA	Positive 1/640	
Anti-dsDNA antibody	Positive	
Anti-Sm antibody	Positive	

Questions

- What are the immediate investigations of choice, and why?
- What is the likely underlying unifying diagnosis, and how would you manage this patient?

ANSWER 66

The patient's current history and examination findings are consistent with pericarditis, a pericardial effusion (with possible cardiac tamponade) and pleural effusions. The immediate investigations of choice are therefore an ECG and echocardiogram. The ECG in pericarditis classically demonstrates widespread ST segment elevation in a saddle-shaped form; in the presence of a pericardial effusion the complexes may also be small. Echocardiography is critical to assess diastolic filling and guide decisions regarding pericardiocentesis.

The underlying unifying diagnosis is systemic lupus erythematosus (SLE), a multisystem autoimmune condition characterized by antibodies directed against nuclear components. SLE is more common, and more severe, in people of Afro-Caribbean origin and may present with multiple problems affecting skin, mucosa, serosa and internal organs. Constitutional upset and Raynaud's phenomenon are also frequently encountered. The American College of Rheumatology devised classification criteria to assist in recruitment to SLE clinical trials; these are now frequently adopted as diagnostic criteria. Four out of the eleven criteria must be met, either concurrently or sequentially, to make a diagnosis of SLE; the present patient fulfils six of them.

! American College of Rheumatology Classification Criteria for SLE (1997)	
Oral ulcers	Recurrent and often confluent
Malar rash	'Butterfly' rash across cheeks and nose, sparing nasolabial folds
Discoid rash	Discrete lesions with scaling and pigmentation change
Photosensitivity	Exacerbation of rashes and constitutional upset following sun exposure
Arthralgia	Non-erosive, occasional ligamentous laxity (Jaccoud's arthropathy)
Serositis	Pleurisy or pericarditis
Renal disease	Proteinuria or cellular casts
Haematological disease	Leuco- or lymphopenia, haemolytic anaemia, thrombocytopenia
Neurological disease	Seizures or psychosis
Anti-nuclear factor positivity	Positive in >99% of patients
Immunological abnormality	Anti-dsDNA or anti-SM or positive antiphospholipid antibodies

Serological indicators of active SLE include the following.

- There is an elevated ESR. The CRP, however, is classically normal, unless there is serosal (i.e. pleuropericardial) involvement – as in this case. In the absence of clear serosal involvement, an elevated CRP in a lupus patient should prompt a search for infection.
- There is low complement (C3 and/or C4 counts) due to immune complex consumption.
- dsDNA titres in some patients mimic disease activity and a rapid rise in titre may predate a clinical flare.

Renal disease remains the most feared complication of lupus and all patients (including this one!) should have their blood pressure checked, urine examined for casts and serum creatinine checked regularly.

The management of lupus depends on disease activity. For the majority with mild disease, simple measures such as avoiding sun exposure and using NSAIDs for mild arthralgia are sufficient. For those with moderate disease, hydroxychloroquine, steroids and steroid-sparing agents such as methotrexate or azathioprine are appropriate; but those with organ-threatening disease will require more powerful immunosuppression in the form of cyclophosphamide or mycophenolate mofetil. The anti-B-cell monoclonal antibody rituximab may also be useful in refractory disease. This patient has significant serosal and haematological involvement so would need a course of steroids to get the disease under control before commencing a steroid-sparing agent. If her urine dip and/or creatinine indicate renal disease, a renal biopsy should be considered to guide decisions regarding further immunosuppression.

 KEY POINTS

- SLE is a classic autoimmune disease.
- Anti-nuclear factor is sensitive but not specific: a negative result in screening investigations is therefore reassuring.
- Since renal involvement is the most feared complication, all lupus patients should have their blood pressure and renal function checked, along with a urine dip to look for haematuria.

CASE 67: PAINFUL HANDS AND BREATHLESSNESS

History

A 36-year-old woman is referred by her general practitioner with cold, painful hands and shortness of breath on exertion. Over the last 6 weeks she has noticed her fingers and hands turning blue, then white and finally red and painful in episodic attacks, particularly in the cold. In addition the skin on her fingers feels taut, reducing her ability to make a fist. The shortness of breath and reduced exercise tolerance has developed insidiously over the same period but she has not had a cough or infective symptoms. She has no history of, or risk factors for, respiratory disease.

Examination

This woman is dyspnoeic on walking from the waiting room to the clinic; her oxygen saturations are initially 92 per cent but increase to 99 per cent with rest. She has no peripheral stigmata of respiratory disease. The skin over her fingers and hands is tight and bound-down but is intact with no evidence of ulcers or vasculitis. The thickened skin extends beyond her elbows and she also has restricted mouth opening. Her jugular venous pulse is elevated, with a parasternal heave and a loud second heart sound, but there is no peripheral oedema. In the respiratory system she has bibasal mid-to-late fine inspiratory crackles.

Questions

- What is the cause of this patient's breathlessness and cardiorespiratory findings?
- What is the underlying diagnosis?
- What are the possible complications?
- How would you further investigate and manage this patient?

ANSWER 67

This woman has the clinical features of interstitial lung disease (progressive breathlessness, desaturation on exercise and typical crackles) and is developing right heart failure (raised JVP, right ventricular heave and loud P2) as a result. The colour changes in her hands are a very good description of triphasic Raynaud's phenomenon: episodic vasospasm that may be primary (idiopathic) or secondary due to an underlying connective tissue disease. The combination of Raynaud's phenomenon, skin tightening and interstitial lung disease would strongly suggest an underlying diagnosis of scleroderma in this case.

Scleroderma is an uncommon disorder characterized by thickening of the skin and, to a greater or lesser degree, fibrosis of internal organs. The condition is classified according to the extent of disease.

Localized scleroderma is restricted to the skin with no evidence of internal organ involvement. Patterns of limited disease occur as isolated fibrotic plaques (morphoea) or bands of affected skin (linear scleroderma, also known as 'en coup de sabre' when found on the face).

Systemic sclerosis is divided into diffuse and limited forms.

* Diffuse systemic sclerosis is characterized by fibrosis extending proximal to elbows or knees. These patients are likely to describe recent-onset Raynaud's phenomenon and are at greater risk of developing cardiopulmonary, renal or gastrointestinal complications. Typically they have anti-topoisomerase-1 (anti-Scl70) antibodies.
* Limited systemic sclerosis results in distal fibrotic skin disease. The associated Raynaud's phenomenon tends to be longstanding and these patients are more likely to develop telangiectasias, calcinosis and pulmonary hypertension. The characteristic antibody profile is anti-centromere positivity.

! Potential systemic involvement in scleroderma	
Vasomotor	Raynaud's phenomenon
Cutaneous	Thickening, telangiectasias, calcinosis, microstomia
Musculoskeletal	Tendon friction rubs, myopathy, osteolysis, arthralgia (but erosive arthritis rare)
Gastrointestinal	Oesophageal dysmotility, diminished peristalsis and bacterial overgrowth
Cardiovascular	Pulmonary hypertension
Respiratory	Interstitial lung disease
Renal	Renal crisis with hypertension, microangiopathic haemolysis

Although this patient almost certainly has diffuse systemic sclerosis, the diagnosis should be confirmed serologically with an antibody screen (ANA, antiScl-70 and anti-centromere). The extent of internal organ involvement should be ascertained by checking renal function and making a full assessment of her respiratory system. Appropriate investigations would include an X-ray and high-resolution CT scan of her chest, along with pulmonary function to assess lung volumes and gas transfer. Echocardiography will determine the presence and severity of pulmonary hypertension and right heart failure.

There is no specific treatment for systemic sclerosis. Raynaud's phenomenon is managed by keeping warm and using vasodilators such as nifedipine. Interstitial lung disease may respond to immunosuppression with steroids and cyclophosphamide. Right heart failure is managed with diuretic therapy. The risk of developing renal crisis is diminished by the use of prophylactic angiotensin-converting enzyme (ACE) inhibition.

 KEY POINTS

- Scleroderma is characterized by skin thickening and a variable extent of internal organ involvement.
- Limited disease is not necessarily more benign as a significant proportion develop pulmonary disease.

CASE 68: PERSISTENT ULCERATION IN AN ELDERLY WOMAN

History

A 78-year-old woman is referred from a leg-ulcer clinic to rheumatology for advice. She has been treated with compression bandaging for presumed venous ulcers for several months, with no perceptible benefit, and on a recent review was found to have a few scattered lesions of palpable purpura, an elevated ESR and a very high rheumatoid factor.

Examination

This woman has palpable purpura over her feet and toes, with a shallow painful ulcer on her left shin and one over her right first metatarsophalangeal (MTP) joint. The edges of the ulcers are punched out but not heaped up, and the bases are clean with no evidence of infection. There is no clinical evidence of synovitis and the remainder of the examination is normal.

INVESTIGATIONS		
		Normal range
Haemoglobin	14.9 g/dL	13.3–17.7 g/dL
White cell count	7.4×10^9/L	$3.9–10.6 \times 10^9$/L
Platelets	435×10^9/L	$150–440 \times 10^9$/L
ESR	104 mm/h	<10 mm/h
Rheumatoid factor	985 iU/mL	<11 iU/mL
C3	41 mg/dL	65–190 mg/dL
C4	8 mg/dL	14–40 mg/dL

Questions

- What is the diagnosis?
- What are potential complications?
- How would you further investigate and manage this patient?

ANSWER 68

Palpable purpura may occur in conditions such as meningococcal sepsis and thrombocytopenic purpura, but one of the most common inflammatory causes of palpable purpura is vasculitis. Although all of the small to medium vessel vasculitides can give rise to purpura, the most common underlying conditions are Henoch–Schönlein purpura, leucocytoclastic vasculitis and cryoglobulinaemia.

Cryoglobulins are immunoglobulins or immunoglobulin complexes that precipitate out in the cold. Some cryoglobulins have rheumatoid factor activity, giving rise to a very high RF titre in the absence of rheumatoid arthritis – as in this case. The complement is consumed during immune complex formation, giving rise to low serum levels of C3 and C4.

Cryoglobulinaemias exist in single and mixed forms.

- A single homogeneous form (25 per cent), also known as type I, can be essential or idiopathic, but is often associated with myeloma, lymphoma or Waldenström's macroglobulinaemia.
- The mixed form (75 per cent) is further subdivided into mixed monoclonal (type II) and polyclonal (type III), and both types may form complexes with self IgG (i.e. have rheumatoid factor activity). Although the mixed cryoglobulinaemias can be essential, type II is often associated with myeloma, lymphoma, Sjögren's syndrome and infections (particularly hepatitis C). Type III is classically associated with autoimmune inflammatory disease (particularly RA and SLE).

The complications of cryoglobulinaemia are classically cutaneous with palpable purpura, petechiae, distal ulceration/necrosis and livedo seen most commonly. Other common features to look out for are Raynaud's phenomenon, arthritis, peripheral neuropathy and renal disease. As renal involvement is the greatest predictor of outcome, this patient should have her renal function and blood pressure checked, along with a urine dip checking for proteinuria or haematuria. Liver disease is present in up to 70 per cent due to the association between hepatitis C infection and type II cryoglobulinaemia, so hepatitis C serology should be checked in all patients with a suspected small to medium vessel vasculitis.

Cryoglobulin levels themselves are diagnostic, but measuring them can be technically challenging as significant quantities are lost when the blood cools to below 37°C. Either the blood should be drawn in the department where the testing is to take place or steps be taken to incubate the blood during transfer to the laboratory.

Treatment of cryoglobulinaemia depends on the extent of disease and the association with hepatitis C. For those with no evidence of hepatitis, treatment consists of cold avoidance, non-steroidal anti-inflammatory drugs (NSAIDs) and hydroxychloroquine, escalating to corticosteroids and steroid-sparing agents such as azathioprine if necessary. Cytotoxic therapy (cyclophosphamide) or plasmapharesis is reserved for those with organ or life-threatening disease. For patients with hepatitis-associated disease, the treatment of choice is interferon-α with or without the antiviral ribavirin; these may have to be combined with immunosuppressive agents if the vasculitis is very severe.

KEY POINTS

- Cryoglobulins are immunoglobulins (or complexes thereof) that precipitate out in the cold.
- Consider cryoglobulins in patients with palpable purpura and skin ulceration.
- The most common mixed forms have rheumatoid factor activity and may produce a very high RF titre.
- Testing for cryoglobulins requires the sample to reach the lab at 37°C!

CASE 69: A SORE THROAT, PAINFUL KNEES AND FACIAL MOVEMENTS

History

A 16-year-old boy is referred to the medical team with abnormal involuntary facial movements. He was well until 8 weeks before admission when he developed a sore throat and febrile illness, associated with pain and swelling in several large joints. The symptoms began in his knees, before moving to his ankles and finally his elbows and responded only partially to ibuprofen. However, he made a full recovery within 3 weeks. For the last 24 hours his parents have noticed emotional lability and involuntary rapid and purposeless movements, particularly in his face. He denies weakness or sensory loss.

Examination

This adolescent is well and not febrile. He has brief uncoordinated facial movements consistent with chorea. His skin, nails and mucosal surfaces are normal. Cardiovascular examination reveals a friction rub and pansystolic murmur in the mitral area. Respiratory and abdominal examinations are normal. There is a cool effusion in his left elbow.

Questions

- What is the likely diagnosis?
- What investigations would you request?
- What are the treatment options?

ANSWER 69

The combination of a sore throat and febrile illness in a young person followed by a migratory polyarthropathy, chorea and carditis is highly suggestive of rheumatic fever. This systemic connective tissue disease occurs typically between 3 and 10 weeks after the original group A streptococcal infection and, as in this case, chorea is often the most delayed manifestation.

The diagnosis is made on the basis of the Duckett Jones criteria: two minor or one major plus two minor criteria are required, plus supporting evidence of preceding group A streptococcal infection, such as elevated ASOT (see the box).

! Duckett Jones criteria (1944)	
Major criteria	
Pancarditis	Endocarditis (most commonly mitral and aortic valves)
	Myocarditis (cardiac failure and conduction defects)
	Pericarditis
Polyarthritis	Migratory large-joint arthropathy
(Sydenham's) Chorea	May be associated with emotional lability
Erythema marginatum	Erythematous rings on trunk and inside of limbs
Subcutaneous nodules	Firm, painless, may resolve rapidly
Minor criteria	
Arthralgia	
Fever	
Elevated ESR/CRP	
Prolonged PR interval	
Previous rheumatic fever	

The arthritis associated with rheumatic fever classically involves the large joints (knees, ankles, elbows and wrists) and occurs in up to three-quarters of patients. It is mild, non-erosive and self-limiting, tending to resolve within 2–4 weeks.

The investigations of choice begin with an echocardiogram to assess valvular insufficiency and to identify a pericardial effusion. The specific antibody test used to help confirm a diagnosis of rheumatic fever is the antistreptolysin-O (ASO) and elevated titres (>200 units) are found in up to 80 per cent of patients with rheumatic fever, although high ASO titres may also be found in patients with other rheumatic diseases. Other possible, non-specific features of rheumatic fever include an elevated acute-phase response (ESR/CRP), a normocytic anaemia, neutrophilia and hypoalbuminaemia.

Treatment is with penicillin (or erythromycin in those with penicillin sensitivity); the inflammatory component of disease is treated with salicylates or, in the case of severe disease, corticosteroids. Those with a history of confirmed rheumatic fever are at lifetime risk of developing recurrent disease with subsequent streptococcal infection and should receive secondary prophylaxis in the form of continuous penicillin for 5 years or until 21 years of age, whichever is longer.

🔑 KEY POINTS
• Rheumatic fever may occur following streptococcal infection.
• Cardinal features are arthritis, carditis, rashes and chorea (a late sign).
• Penicillin is the treatment of choice. Corticosteroids may be required for the inflammatory symptoms.

CASE 70: A LUMPY RASH AND A SWOLLEN KNEE

History

A 24-year-old woman is referred by her general practitioner with a rash over the front of her shins and an intermittently swollen knee. There is no relevant medical history. She is a non-smoker who drinks around 8 units of alcohol per week and is taking no medication except vitamin pills bought over the counter in a health food shop. Her mother has type 2 diabetes. She works as a teacher.

Examination

The lesions over this young woman's shins are raised and tender. They are of differing ages and sizes, between 5 and 20 mm, passing through the stages of a bruise as they fade. There are no other skin lesions. Although she reports knee swelling in the past, there is no current evidence of inflammatory arthropathy.

Questions

- What is the rash?
- What management would be appropriate?

ANSWER 70

The description of the rash is typical of erythema nodosum. This is most common over the shins although it may occasionally be seen over the arms or thighs. Common causes for erythema nodosum include:

- pregnancy
- inflammatory bowel disease
- sarcoidosis
- tuberculosis
- streptococcal infection
- drugs (sulphonamides, penicillin, oral contraceptives among others)
- Behçet's syndrome
- rheumatic fever
- idiopathic.

The history should be directed towards highlighting or eliminating these most common underlying conditions by seeking out their associated symptoms. Direct questions in the systems review might therefore include: pregnancy or contraceptive pill use; fever, sore throat, cough or breathlessness; diarrhoea or abdominal pain; presence and pattern of arthropathy. A detailed drug history is also mandatory.

Mild idiopathic erythema nodosum (as in this case) needs no specific treatment. If the rash is troublesome, a non-steroidal anti-inflammatory drug (NSAID) or, if severe, corticosteroids are effective. Any underlying condition is treated independently of the rash.

 KEY POINTS

- The rash of erythema nodosum is raised, tender lumps over the shins which discolour like a bruise.
- It often does not require any specific treatment. Screening questions should be directed at eliminating an associated underlying condition.

CASE 71: RASH AND SWOLLEN ANKLES

History

A 28-year-old woman presents with a 3-day history of a facial rash and swelling of her ankles. She has never had a rash before, has not changed her facial cream or been exposed to anything that might precipitate an allergic reaction. The swelling of the ankles coincided with the development of the rash. Initially it was mild with 'sock-marks' around her ankles, but now the swelling is more pronounced and has spread up to her knees. She is otherwise well and on no medication.

Examination

This young woman has a maculopapular rash across the bridge of her nose and cheeks with sparing of the nasolabial folds. There is pitting oedema of the lower limbs to just above the knee. She is hypertensive at 154/90 mmHg, but the remainder of the examination is normal.

INVESTIGATIONS		
		Normal range
Haemoglobin	14.2 g/dL	13.3–17.7 g/dL
White cell count	3.6×10^9/L	$3.9–10.6 \times 10^9$/L
Platelets	367×10^9/L	$150–440 \times 10^9$/L
ESR	76 mm/h	<10 mm/h
CRP	<5 mg/L	<5 mg/L
Urea	15.2 mmol/L	2.5–6.7 mmol/L
Creatinine	168 µmol/L	70–120 µmol/L
Albumin	27 g/L	35–50 g/L
ANA	1/640	
Anti-dsDNA	Detected	
C3	52 mg/dL	65–190 mg/dL
C4	6 mg/dL	14–40 mg/dL
Urine dipstick	3+ blood, 3+ protein	

Questions

- What is the likely diagnosis?
- How would you further investigate and manage this patient?

ANSWER 71

This patient has lupus nephritis and needs urgent referral to renal services for consideration of a renal biopsy and then potent immunosuppression. The diagnosis of lupus is suggested by the combination of:

- classic malar rash
- leucopenia
- positive anti-nuclear factor
- positive dsDNA antibodies
- renal disease (elevated urea and creatinine, proteinuria and haematuria and hypertension).

Renal biopsies are performed both for diagnosis and to aid prognostication. Lupus damages the kidneys by immune complex deposition – hence the low complement levels in this patient, as they have been consumed. This can be observed with immunofluorescence studies of glomerular tissue. In addition, the biopsy will give an indication of how much of the disease is acute (and therefore reversible) and how much damage is chronic and non-salvageable.

Treatment of lupus nephritis focuses on tight control of blood pressure with an angiotensin-converting enzyme (ACE) inhibitor and powerful immunosuppression. All patients should receive high-dose steroids (up to 1 mg/kg) and either cyclophosphamide or mycophenolate mofetil. Both drugs are effective in this situation; but, as this patient is of child-bearing age, mycophenolate mofetil may be preferable as cyclophosphamide has an adverse effect on fertility. If the patient fails to respond to treatment, anti-B-cell therapy or plasma exchange are alternative therapeutic options.

 KEY POINTS

- Renal disease is the most feared complication of SLE.
- Renal biopsy is used to guide treatment and aids prognostication.
- Most patients will require potent immunosuppression.
- Cyclophosphamide reduces fertility and this side-effect should be specifically discussed with patients of child-bearing age.

CASE 72: A BREATHLESS RHEUMATOID PATIENT

History

A 46-year-old man with rheumatoid arthritis attends an emergency review at his rheumatology department. His joint disease is well-controlled on methotrexate 20 mg/week. Over the last few weeks, however, he has become increasingly short of breath with a marked reduction in exercise tolerance. He has a dry, unproductive cough and, although he denies infective symptoms, he recalls feeling feverish at the beginning of his illness. He is a non-smoker and there is no relevant occupational history.

Examination

This man is mildly short of breath at rest (18 breaths per minute). He is not febrile. Oxygen saturation is 98 per cent on room air, desaturating rapidly to 88 per cent on exercise. Breath sounds are heard throughout both lung fields, with late inspiratory fine crackles bibasally. A radiograph is shown in Fig. 72.1.

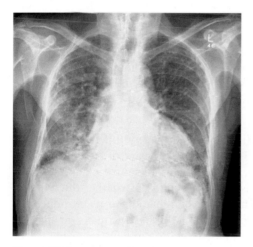

Figure 72.1

Questions

- What is the differential diagnosis?
- What other investigations should be done?

ANSWER 72

 Differential diagnosis for a breathless rheumatoid patient

- Rheumatoid lung: interstitial lung disease, generally a non-specific interstitial pneumonitis
- Drug reaction causing allergic alveolitis: classically reported for methotrexate
- Coexistent infection: bacterial or pneumocystis pneumonia, particularly in the immunosuppressed and patients on steroids
- Pleural effusion: exudate with high LDH and low glucose
- Bronchiolitis obliterans

The chest X-ray reveals widespread but predominantly bibasal interstitial shadowing. Further investigation of this particular patient should aim to differentiate between interstitial lung disease, methotrexate lung and coexistent infection. Bronchopneumonia is unlikely given the lack of fever, sputum and features of consolidation, but PCP (pneumocystis pneumonia) may present in this way.

In terms of simple investigations, a full blood count can be very helpful. The FBC is classically normal in interstitial lung disease, but there may be an elevated white cell count in infection and methotrexate reactions tend to be associated with an eosinophilia. The C-reactive protein may be very elevated in bacterial infection (although make sure that active inflammatory joint disease is not contributing to this). Special investigations are very helpful in this case: lung function tests and a high-resolution CT of the chest are investigations of choice.

Methotrexate lung is an idiosyncratic reaction (i.e. may occur at any time after introduction of the drug) but occurs more commonly in the first 2–3 years of treatment. Most cases resolve on cessation of the drug, but occasionally a short course of oral steroids may accelerate resolution of the attack. There is very little data on whether the reaction recurs on re-challenge, but most rheumatologists would be reluctant to re-introduce the offending drug, even at a lower dose. Rheumatoid lung is harder to treat and may be rapidly progressive (Hamman–Rich syndrome). In cases with radiological evidence of active inflammation in the form of ground-glass shadowing rather than clear-cut fibrosis, immunosuppression with steroids and cyclophosphamide may be appropriate. These patients should be discussed with respiratory units with expertise in interstitial lung disease.

🔑 | **KEY POINTS**

- Breathlessness in rheumatoid patients is a common clinical problem.
- The key differential diagnoses are rheumatoid lung, infection or drug reaction (alveolitis).
- Close liaison with respiratory units is important.

CASE 73: PLEURITIC CHEST PAIN

History

A 38-year-old patient presents to the emergency department with acute pleuritic chest pain and breathlessness. She denies cough, infective symptoms or risk factors for deep venous thrombosis. She is otherwise well. Her medical history includes lupus erythematosus which is currently in remission, and a second-trimester miscarriage.

Examination

This woman is uncomfortable and short of breath at rest with a respiratory rate of 16 breaths per minute. Her pulse is 96/min sinus rhythm, blood pressure 115/68 mmHg, and oxygen saturation 90 per cent on room air. She is not febrile. The remainder of her clinical examination is normal. A radiograph is shown in Fig. 73.1.

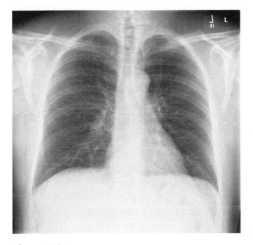

Figure 73.1

🔍 INVESTIGATIONS		
		Normal range
Haemoglobin	14.9 g/dL	13.3–17.7 g/dL
White cell count	5.6 × 10⁹/L	3.9–10.6 × 10⁹/L
Platelets	98 × 10⁹/L	150–440 × 10⁹/L

Questions
- What is the likely cause of this patient's chest pain and breathlessness?
- What is the diagnostic test for this?
- Is the history of lupus relevant?

ANSWER 73

The likely diagnosis for this patient's current presentation is pulmonary embolus (PE). The history of sudden-onset pleuritic chest pain and shortness of breath is characteristic of PE, and the normal respiratory examination and chest X-ray is highly supportive, as is the hypoxia. Although an ECG may demonstrate right heart strain in patients with large emboli, the most common finding is simply a sinus tachycardia (or new-onset atrial fibrillation in the elderly). The diagnostic test for PE is a CT–pulmonary angiogram (CT-PA) and the patient should be anticoagulated in anticipation of a positive result. The history of lupus is highly relevant and, in combination with a previous pregnancy loss and mild thrombocytopenia, raises the possibility of antiphospholipid syndrome.

Antiphospholipid syndrome is a hypercoagulable state characterized by recurrent arteriovenous thrombosis and/or pregnancy morbidity in the presence of either a lupus anticoagulant or anticardiolipin antibody (both phospholipid-related proteins). The term 'lupus anticoagulant' is admittedly confusing in a pro-thrombotic state, but the in-vitro test relies on prolonged coagulation (APTT) that is corrected not by addition of a clotting factor but rather by the addition of phospholipid in excess. Although antiphospholipid syndrome was originally described in lupus, its occurrence does not correlate with disease activity and it may indeed occur in patients with no clinical or serological evidence of SLE.

The most common arteriovenous thrombotic events in antiphospholipid syndrome are deep venous thrombosis and pulmonary embolus (as in this case), but any part of the circulation may be involved, with arterial events such as myocardial infarction and stroke carrying a high mortality rate. Poor placental circulation is thought to be responsible for the high pregnancy morbidity, with recurrent first- and second-trimester loss and a higher rate of pre-eclampsia being typical clinical features. The Sapporo criteria for the diagnosis of antiphospholipid syndrome require one clinical and one laboratory criterion to be fulfilled; the laboratory criteria need to be met twice at least 6 weeks apart.

! | **Sapporo criteria for the diagnosis of antiphospholipid syndrome**

Clinical criteria	*Laboratory criteria*
Arterial or venous thrombosis	Anticardiolipin antibodies
Obstetric loss:	Lupus anticoagulant
3 or more miscarriages before 10 weeks gestation	
1 or more miscarriage after 10 weeks gestation	
1 or more premature delivery (<34 weeks) due to pre-eclampsia	

Additional clinical features may include:

• cardiac valvular disease (up to a third have mitral valve prolapse)
• livedo reticularis
• mild chronic thrombocytopenia
• neurological disease such as chorea or transverse myelitis.

Management of antiphospholipid syndrome is lifetime anticoagulation with warfarin, typically aiming for an INR of 2.0–3.0. All patients should be advised to stop smoking. Special attention should be paid to primary prevention of atheromatous disease with aggressive blood pressure, cholesterol and diabetes management. Oestrogen-containing contraceptives and hormone replacement therapy are contraindicated in women with antiphospholipid syndrome. Anticoagulation during pregnancy can be a challenge as warfarin is teratogenic and must be stopped before 6 weeks' gestation. However, with specialist obstetric care and the combination of low-dose aspirin plus low-molecular-weight heparin, the rate of successful pregnancies has increased considerably.

 KEY POINTS

- Antiphospholipid syndrome may occur independently of SLE.
- Recurrent miscarriage is a frequent clinical feature.
- Diagnostic tests are anticardiolipin antibodies and antiphospholipid antibodies.

CASE 74: FEVER, RASH AND JOINT PAINS

History

A 28-year-old man is admitted to the infectious diseases unit with pyrexia of unknown origin. For the last 10 weeks he has been feeling non-specifically unwell with joint pains, muscle aches and weight loss. During this time he has had a recurrent fever, occasionally very high (>40°C) which has not responded to multiple courses of antibiotics. Of note, the fever spikes only once or twice a day, usually in the morning or late afternoon; in between febrile episodes his temperature is normal and he feels reasonably well. In addition he has noticed a faint rash over his trunk which is most evident when he has a temperature. During the course of his illness many of his joints have been painful and stiff, and currently his knees, wrists and the small joints of his hands are worst affected.

Examination

This young man appears unwell but is not febrile. There is a very faint salmon-pink rash over his abdomen and lymphadenopathy in the cervical and axillary regions. Cardiorespiratory examination is unremarkable. There is two-fingers breadth hepatomegaly but his spleen is impalpable. Musculoskeletal examination reveals widespread mild synovitis in his hands and wrists and an effusion in his left knee.

🔍 **INVESTIGATIONS**

		Normal range
Haemoglobin	10.2 g/dL	13.3–17.7 g/dL
Mean corpuscular volume (MCV)	85 fL	80–99 fL
White cell count	22.3×10^9/L	$3.9–10.6 \times 10^9$/L
Platelets	642×10^9/l	$150–440 \times 10^9$/L
ESR	95 mm/h	<10 mm/h
CRP	>160 mg/L	<5 mg/L
Anti-nuclear factor	Negative	
Rheumatoid factor	Negative	
Blood cultures (3 sets)	No growth after 5 days	

Questions
- What is the differential diagnosis?
- What is the most likely diagnosis?
- What blood test might aid diagnosis?
- What is the treatment of choice?

ANSWER 74

The differential diagnosis in this situation is wide. Many of the features are relatively non-specific, and the blood tests simply reveal evidence of marked systemic inflammation in the absence of clear bacterial infection or seropositivity. Diagnoses to consider include:

- infection
- lymphoma
- leukaemia
- sarcoidosis
- endocarditis
- rheumatic fever.

However, the presence of the swinging daily (quotidian) rather than persistent fever with spikes and the evanescent rash are characteristic of adult-onset Still's disease – a systemic inflammatory illness associated with a seronegative chronic polyarthropathy.

The most common features of adult-onset Still's disease are:

- arthralgia ± arthritis
- characteristic fever
- myalgias
- rash
- weight loss
- lymphadenopathy
- hepatosplenomegaly
- abdominal pain
- serositis (pleuropericarditis).

There is no diagnostic test for Still's disease and often there is considerable delay as patients undergo several negative investigations. However, an extremely elevated ferritin (often >1000 mg/dL) is highly suggestive of the diagnosis and would certainly be an investigation of choice in this case.

The treatment of choice is corticosteroid therapy, the dose of which is increased in line with the severity of the patient's illness. Many – this case included – may require doses of up to 60 mg/day initially to get the disease under control before adding in a steroid-sparing agent such as methotrexate to aid gradual steroid withdrawal.

Generally, patients with adult-onset Still's disease fall into one of three categories: self-limiting illness, intermittent flares of disease activity, or chronic arthritis. The overall survival rate at 5 years is 90–95 per cent.

 KEY POINTS

- Consider inflammatory disease in cases of pyrexia of unknown origin.
- The quotidian rash is characteristic of adult-onset Still's disease.
- The serum ferritin is markedly elevated in Still's disease.

CASE 75: PAIN AND STIFFNESS IN SHOULDERS AND HIPS

History

A 72-year-old woman presents to her general practitioner with a few weeks' history of pain and stiffness affecting her shoulders and hips. The pain began insidiously but is now severe; her shoulders and neck are worst and affected symmetrically. Although she denies objective weakness, the pain is limiting her activities of daily living and frequently wakes her from sleep. The stiffness lasts several hours in the morning. Otherwise, she is entirely well and has no medical history of note.

Examination

This elderly woman is uncomfortable and finds it difficult to move from the chair to the examining couch. She is generally tender around the neck, shoulders and pelvic girdle. There is no evidence of synovitis but full range of movement is limited by periarticular rather than true joint pain.

INVESTIGATIONS		
		Normal range
Haemoglobin	14.2 g/dL	13.3–17.7 g/dL
White cell count	9.3×10^9/L	$3.9–10.6 \times 10^9$/L
Platelets	242×10^9/L	$150–440 \times 10^9$/L
ESR	45 mm/h	<10 mm/h
CRP	69 mg/L	<5 mg/L

Questions

- What is the most likely diagnosis?
- What is the differential diagnosis and screening tests?
- What is the most significant complication?

ANSWER 75

The most likely diagnosis is polymyalgia rheumatica (PMR), a systemic inflammatory syndrome affecting the elderly that is characterized by bilateral pain and stiffness in the shoulders and hip girdles. The stiffness can be profound and limits mobility although true muscle weakness is not a feature. Physical examination is essentially unremarkable, although patients with a marked constitutional upset due to PMR may appear unwell with evidence of recent weight loss. The affected areas are diffusely tender, with movements limited by pain. Synovitis has been reported, but care must be taken not to attribute joint inflammation to PMR until other diagnoses have been excluded; for example, a significant minority of RA patients may present with a polymyalgic onset.

The acute-phase response (classically ESR) is elevated in PMR, although can be normal in a minority of cases; the diagnosis of PMR is a clinical one, and further investigations are 'screening tests', performed to exclude alternative diagnoses.

! Differential diagnosis of polymyalgia rheumatica	
Rheumatoid arthritis	Small-joint arthropathy – the majority RF or ACPA positive
Infection	Fevers or localizing symptoms and signs, blood cultures may be positive
Malignancy	Atypical presentation, suggestive features in history or examination, poor response to therapy, investigations guided by history and examination
Polymyositis	Muscle weakness, elevated CK, abnormal EMG or MRI findings
Fibromyalgia	Trigger points and normal ESR and CRP
Hypothyroidism	Stigmata of thyroid disease, elevated TSH, normal ESR and CRP
Depression	Normal physical examination, normal ESR and CRP

The treatment for PMR is low-dose corticosteroids. Prednisolone 15 mg daily should suffice, but may have to be increased according to weight. Many physicians would consider a dramatic response to low-dose predisolone as almost diagnostic for PMR, so if a patient's symptoms do not improve rapidly it is wise to re-evaluate the original diagnosis. Most patients will successfully wean down and off steroids over 18 months or 2 years, but if dose reduction is a problem, steroid-sparing agents such as methotrexate may be beneficial. All patients should receive concomitant bone protection with their corticosteroids.

The most significant complication of PMR is the development of an associated temporal (giant cell) arteritis, a granulomatous large-vessel vasculitis which may, if untreated, lead to blindness. Any patient with a history of PMR should be assessed with this in mind and asked to report any history of headaches, scalp tenderness or visual disturbance. Diagnosing temporal arteritis is difficult; it is based on a combination of the clinical picture, an elevated acute-phase response and histological features on temporal artery biopsy.

 KEY POINTS

- Polymyalgia rheumatica is common and responds very swiftly to low-dose corticosteroid therapy.
- The feared association is temporal (giant cell) arteritis, which may lead to blindness.

CASE 76: PAINFUL EARS AND NOSE

History

A 50-year-old man presents to his general practitioner with attacks of painful ears and tenderness across the nasal bridge, which has begun to collapse. During each episode, his ears feel swollen, 'like they're burning', and hot to touch; the bridge of his nose feels full and painful, with occasional nose-bleeds. During this current attack, his ears and nasal bridge have started to feel floppy. Otherwise he is well, with no past medical history of note.

Examination

Both ears are tender and hot to touch, with boggy swelling and a purplish discoloration. The earlobes are spared. His nasal bridge has collapsed, causing a saddle-nose deformity. His right eye has an injected sclera and there is asymmetric polyarthritis affecting his hands. The remainder of the examination is normal.

INVESTIGATIONS		
		Normal range
Haemoglobin	15.2 g/dL	13.3–17.7 g/dL
White cell count	9.1×10^9/L	$3.9–10.6 \times 10^9$/L
Platelets	545×10^9/L	$150–440 \times 10^9$/L
ESR	47 mm/h	<10 mm/h
CRP	68 mg/L	<5 mg/L
Immunoglobulins	Polyclonal hypergammaglobulinaemia	

Questions

• What is the differential diagnosis of a saddle-nose deformity?
• What is the diagnosis in this case, and what other associated features might there be?
• How would you manage this patient?

ANSWER 76

The differential diagnosis of a collapsed nasal septum and saddle-nose deformity is:

- relapsing polychondritis
- Wegener's granulomatosis
- congenital syphilis.

The auricular disease in this case is limited to the cartilage as the earlobe is spared. This effectively rules out cellulitis and the most likely cause of such multifocal cartilaginous inflammation is relapsing polychondritis. Relapsing polychondritis is characterized histologically by inflammatory infiltration and later fibrosis of cartilage. Any cartilage, in any location, is at risk, but the box shows classic sites for clinically relevant disease.

! Clinical features of relapsing polychondritis	
Auricular disease	Attacks of painful inflammation Development of 'cauliflower ear'
Nasal chondritis	Painful nasal fullness Epistaxis Nasal septal collapse
Arthritis	Generally oligo- or polyarticular Non-erosive
Ocular disease	Episcleritis Conjunctivitis Uveitis
Respiratory tract	Throat tenderness Hoarseness Stridor Tracheal stenosis
Audiovestibular	Conductive hearing loss Tinnitus Vertigo
Cardiovascular	Aortic root dilatation
Associated conditions	Systemic vasculitis Glomerulonephritis Systemic lupus erythematosus Rheumatoid arthritis and other rheumatological conditions Myelodysplasia

Diagnosis of relapsing polychondritis is clinical as there are no diagnostic tests – the results of investigations in this case are typical. The ESR can be used as a predictor of disease activity in some patients.

Treatment of relapsing polychondritis is with corticosteroids, the dose of which (20–60 mg/day) depends on the severity of organ involvement and risk to major structures. The majority of patients will need a protracted course of steroids, so steroid-sparing agents should be considered at an early stage and bone protection is mandatory. Surgical reconstruction of collapsed structures is not an option as the deformity tends to continue postoperatively.

KEY POINTS

- Relapsing polychondritis is a cause of painful ears, but the lobe is characteristically spared, differentiating it from cellulitis.
- Any cartilaginous structure may be affected.

CASE 77: WEAKNESS AND A RASH

History

A 72-year-old woman is admitted by the medical team with muscle weakness and pain. Her symptoms began insidiously over the last few weeks, but are now so severe she finds it hard to climb stairs or raise her arms above her head. Fine movements and grip strength are unaffected. She has also noticed a scaly rash over the back of her hands and her palms are becoming cracked and unsightly. Otherwise she is well, with no medical history of note. Systems review is unremarkable; she denies weight loss and in fact has noticed that her abdomen is mildly swollen.

Examination

This elderly woman has marked proximal weakness, graded 2 to 3 out of 5 at shoulder and hip in the absence of neurological features. She has a lilac discolouration over the back of her eyes, a scaly rash on the back of her fingers and papules over her metacarpophalangeal (MCP) joints. Her palms are fissured and cracked and nail-beds are ragged with dilated nail-fold capillary loops. Cardiorespiratory examination is unremarkable. Abdominal examination reveals a non-tender pelvic mass and a small amount of ascites.

INVESTIGATIONS		
		Normal range
Haemoglobin	14.2 g/dL	13.3–17.7 g/dL
White cell count	8.2×10^9/L	$3.9–10.6 \times 10^9$/L
Platelets	342×10^9/L	$150–440 \times 10^9$/L
Creatine kinase	3542 iU/L	25–195 iU/L
ESR	45 mm/h	<10 mm/h
ANA	Positive 1:640	

Questions

- What is the differential diagnosis of this patient's muscle weakness?
- What is the diagnosis in this case?
- How would you further investigate and manage this patient?

ANSWER 77

This elderly woman has a clear-cut proximal myopathy, with a classic history of insidious loss of strength affecting large muscle groups at the shoulder and girdle. The differential diagnosis is broad.

! Differential diagnosis of proximal myopathy	
Inflammatory myopathy	Poly- and dermatomyositis Inclusion body myositis
Drug-induced myopathy	Statins, colchicine, alcohol
Neuromuscular disease	Muscular dystrophies Neuromuscular junction disease (e.g. myasthenia gravis)
Endocrine disease	Hypo- and hyperthyroidism Cushing's and Addison's disease Acromegaly
Metabolic disease	Glycogen storage disorders Malabsorption and vitamin D deficiency Electrolyte disturbance (calcium and potassium)
Rheumatic disorders	Polymyalgia rheumatica, fibromyalgia

The association of a proximal myopathy and a rash in this case, however, suggests the diagnosis of dermatomyositis. This is an autoimmune inflammatory myositis and the elevated CK, ESR and ANA are supportive of the diagnosis. The rashes over her face, hands (the lesions over the knuckles are known as Gottron's papules) and palms (so-called mechanic's hands) are also highly characteristic.

The gold standard investigations for inflammatory myopathy are:

- electromyography which demonstrates myopathic (not neuropathic) potentials
- muscle biopsy revealing a chronic inflammatory infiltrate and muscle necrosis (NB inclusion-body myositis characteristically contains red-rimmed vacuoles with beta-amyloid on biopsy).

MRI (T2-weighted and STIR for fat suppression) will reveal areas of oedema and inflammation and may be useful to delineate areas for biopsy and thereby increase diagnostic yield. Further characterization of the clinical syndrome may also be derived from myositis-specific antibodies. For example, patients with anti-Jo-1 antibody are at a greater risk of developing inflammatory lung disease.

Inflammatory myositis is associated with an underlying malignancy in a significant minority of patients (up to 15 per cent) either at or soon after diagnosis. As a consequence, patients should have a thorough history and examination (including breast, pelvis and prostate) performed specifically looking for occult malignancy; the level of screening investigation is hard to stipulate, but a chest X-ray and mammogram would constitute the bare minimum. This patient has signs suggestive of a pelvic malignancy such as ovarian carcinoma and should undergo an urgent CT scan of her pelvis and abdomen.

Inflammatory myositis is generally steroid responsive, although initially high doses (up to 1 mg/kg) are required to get the disease under control before attempting a slow withdrawal. It may take 2–3 years to get patients off steroids, and in many cases steroid-sparing agents such as methotrexate or azathioprine are required. All patients should also receive bone protection, vitamin D and calcium supplementation. Occasionally diagnostic confusion may arise between a flare of inflammatory myositis and the development of steroid myopathy. Helpful investigations at this stage are to repeat the CK and MRI as both will be abnormal in a flare of inflammatory disease and normal in steroid myopathy.

KEY POINTS

- (Dermato)myositis is an inflammatory cause of proximal myopathy.
- In the elderly, it may be associated with malignancy.
- The muscle disease is generally steroid responsive.

CASE 78: DIARRHOEA, RASH AND A STIFF BACK

History

A 41-year-old man presents to the rheumatology department with bloody diarrhoea, ulcers over his shins and a painful, stiff back. Although his back stiffness began more than 5 years ago, he chose to ignore it until recently when, in combination with his other symptoms, he began to struggle to cope at home. His back pain and stiffness are worse in the morning and tend to ease by lunchtime. It has, on occasion, been associated with a painful and swollen right knee. The diarrhoea and leg ulcers began six weeks previously and he is awaiting a gastroenterology outpatient appointment.

Examination

This man has limited spinal movement in all planes with a Schober's test reduced at 19 cm. His right hip is irritable and there is a moderate effusion of the right knee. There are two ulcers over his left shin with shiny yellow bases and red/blue overhanging edges. The remainder of the examination is normal.

INVESTIGATIONS		
		Normal range
Haemoglobin	14.2 g/dL	13.3–17.7 g/dL
White cell count	6.6×10^9/L	$3.9–10.6 \times 10^9$/L
Platelets	379×10^9/L	$150–440 \times 10^9$/L
ESR	28 mm/h	<10 mm/h
CRP	32 mg/L	<5 mg/L

Questions

• What is the likely unifying diagnosis, and how would you confirm it?
• How would you manage this patient?

ANSWER 78

The most common unifying causes of bloody diarrhoea, rash and arthritis would be Reiter's syndrome or enteropathic (i.e. inflammatory bowel disease) arthritis. However, the duration of the diarrhoea and the description of the rash would suggest enteropathic arthritis is the most likely diagnosis.

A seronegative arthritis may develop in up to 15 per cent of patients with any form of inflammatory bowel disease, including ulcerative colitis (UC), Crohn's disease or microscopic and collagenous colitis. The most common clinical presentations are a peripheral arthritis (commonly divided into type I and type II) and spondyloarthritis.

- Type I enteropathic arthritis is an asymmetrical oligoarthritis which follows disease activity in the bowel.
- Type II enteropathic arthritis is symmetrical and polyarticular and runs an independent course to bowel disease. Both forms of peripheral arthritis affect men and women equally.
- Enteropathic spondyloarthropathy also runs an independent course and may pre- or post-date the bowel disease by several years. It is more common in men than women and presents with inflammatory spinal or sacroiliac pain that is very similar to ankylosing spondylitis.

The extra-articular features of enteropathic arthritis are:

- mucocutaneous: oral ulcers, erythema nodosum, pyoderma gangrenosum
- ocular: anterior uveitis
- musculoskeletal: tendinopathy and enthesopathy, hypertrophic osteopathy.

Investigations reveal a non-specific elevated inflammatory response with a negative RF or ANA (although beware, up to 60 per cent of UC patients are pANCA positive!) and HLA-B27 is positive in 50–70 per cent of cases. The investigation of choice is endoscopy to achieve a histological diagnosis of inflammatory bowel disease, and from a musculoskeletal point of view, the patient needs an MRI of the sacroiliac joints and lumbosacral spine to delineate evidence of inflammatory arthritis.

Treatment of enteropathic arthritis is hampered somewhat by the fact that oral NSAIDs may exacerbate inflammatory bowel disease. Available therapies range from localized treatment with intra-articular steroid injections to systemic management with immunosuppressants such as sulphasalazine or anti-TNF-α agents. Interestingly, spinal disease tends not to respond as well to conventional DMARDs as peripheral arthritis.

 KEY POINTS

- The differential diagnosis of diarrhoea and arthritis includes reactive arthritis and enteropathic arthritis.
- Spinal disease in enteropathic arthritis runs an independent course to bowel disease.

CASE 79: HEADACHE AND WEIGHT LOSS

History

A 62-year-old man presents to his general practitioner with headache. The pain focuses over the temporal areas, where his scalp also feels tender such that he finds it painful to lie on his side at night. Over the same period as his headache has developed, he has noticed pain and fatigue in his jaw when chewing his food. He is otherwise 'reasonably well' but has been experiencing pain and stiffness in his shoulders and hips which he has attributed to heavy gardening, and has lost a few kilograms in weight. His past medical history and systems enquiry is unremarkable and he takes no regular medication.

Examination

This man appears well but uncomfortable. He has marked tenderness to even light touch over his temples; his temporal arteries are tender and pulseless bilaterally. Fundoscopy and the rest of his physical examination are normal.

INVESTIGATIONS		
		Normal range
Haemoglobin	14.2 g/dL	13.3–17.7 g/dL
White cell count	6.3 × 10⁹/L	3.9–10.6 × 10⁹/L
Platelets	542 × 10⁹/L	150–440 × 10⁹/L
ESR	65 mm/h	<10 mm/h
CRP	89 mg/L	<5 mg/L

Questions

- What is the diagnosis?
- What is the investigation of choice?
- How would you manage this patient?

ANSWER 79

The diagnosis is giant cell arteritis (GCA). This granulomatous vasculitis predominantly affects patients over the age of 50 years of age and leads to inflammation and possible occlusion of the aorta and its major branches. Cranial GCA is the most frequently reported, with a classic constellation of symptoms, many of which are evident in this case:

- headache
- scalp tenderness
- jaw claudication
- visual disturbance (e.g. diplopia, amaurosis fugax, blindness)
- tissue necrosis (scalp, tongue).

If patients do experience extracranial disease, the symptoms and signs will correspond to the vascular territory involved. For example, mesenteric ischaemia will generate post-prandial abdominal pain while iliac disease will lead to claudication.

Many GCA patients will have a history of polymyalgia rheumatica (PMR), complaining of bilateral shoulder/pelvic girdle pain and stiffness, although marked constitutional upset such as weight loss or fever tends only to occur in patients with GCA rather than uncomplicated PMR.

This patient's examination findings are classic for GCA, with tender, pulseless temporal vessels. If the ciliary branches of the ophthalmic arteries are involved, visual symptoms ensue and fundoscopy may reveal ischaemic optic neuritis or optic atrophy. Standard simple investigations reveal a non-specific inflammatory picture, with an elevated ESR and/or CRP, thrombocytosis and polyclonal hypergammaglobulinaemia. The investigation of choice is a temporal artery biopsy demonstrating a granulomatous inflammation and a disrupted internal elastic lamina or, less commonly, a diffuse and rather less specific lymphocytic infiltrate. The drawback with biopsy as the gold standard investigation is the presence of 'skip lesions' due to patchy involvement of the vessel, leading to difficulties with false negative results. The diagnosis hinges on the complete picture of clinical suspicion, serological and histological abnormalities.

The treatment of GCA is high-dose corticosteroids (1 mg/kg) and this should be commenced without delay in anyone in whom the diagnosis is suspected. This early use of steroids is crucial to reduce the risk of sight loss and will not dramatically reduce the diagnostic yield of a subsequent biopsy. All patients should receive bone protection with bisphosphonates and calcium/vitamin D supplementation, and many will require gastroprotection in the form of a proton-pump inhibitor. If visual symptoms are present there should be close liaison with local ophthalmology services; in these cases aspirin may provide additional benefit and in the rare instance of sudden total blindness, intravenous methylprednisolone has been reported to restore vision if commenced within 24 hours. Patients should remain on high-dose steroids until symptoms, signs and laboratory indices of inflammation have subsided. This can often take several weeks, and thereafter a very gradual reduction of steroids can commence. As with other conditions requiring long-term steroid therapy, methotrexate or other steroid-sparing agents may prove beneficial. Cyclophosphamide is reserved for the minority of patients who fail to respond to steroid therapy.

KEY POINTS

- Temporal (giant cell) arteritis is the most common of the large-vessel vasculitides.
- The feared complication is blindness.
- Steroid treatment should be commenced without waiting for the diagnostic test (temporal artery biopsy).
- Biopsies may lead to false negative results due to skip lesions.

CASE 80: A PAINFUL SWOLLEN HAND FOLLOWING A FRACTURE

History

A 45-year-old woman fell from her horse and sustained a fracture of her distal radius. Although her fracture healed appropriately with immobilization, the patient noticed that once the cast was removed her wrist was sore and stiff. This deteriorated over a number of weeks, such that her whole hand became painful and swollen.

Examination

The pain does not localize to the joints in particular, and indeed the whole hand appears generally hypersensitive. The skin is shiny and purple and disproportionately sweaty compared to the unaffected side.

Questions

- What is the diagnosis?
- What are the appropriate investigations?
- What treatment options are available?

ANSWER 80

This is a classic description of a regional pain syndrome – also known as chronic regional pain syndromes (CRPS) or reflex sympathetic dystrophy. The condition classically occurs after injury and is characterized by the rapid development of extreme pain that is out of proportion to the initiating event and does not follow an anatomical pattern. In addition there is considerable swelling and the skin may display trophic changes, including increased sweating. Vasomotor instability is also recognized.

Appropriate investigations would include C-reactive protein and/or ESR to rule out an underlying inflammatory arthritis. X-ray features very early on in disease are normal. With persistent disease, the most notable findings are soft-tissue swelling and patchy osteopenia.

Thermography is a specialist investigation and has high sensitivity for thermal changes in the affected limb.

Although there is no specific treatment for chronic regional pain syndromes, prolonged rehabilitation with intensive physiotherapy can be very effective. Other treatment options for resistant or severe disease include neuroleptics like gabapentin or local sympathetic nerve blocks.

 KEY POINTS

- Consider CRPS in any patient presenting with an isolated painful limb following injury.
- Trophic changes and vasomotor instability may help to differentiate CRPS from an inflammatory arthritis.

CASE 81: DIARRHOEA AND PAINFUL JOINTS

History

A 52-year-old man presents with a longstanding history of weight loss, diarrhoea and painful, stiff hips and knees. The arthritis developed first, affecting principally his hips and knees but tending to move around. A rheumatoid factor has been checked in the past and was negative, so he felt reassured. The diarrhoea then became an issue over the last 6 months; he has intermittent abdominal pain and complains that the stools are foul-smelling and hard to flush away. There has never been any blood, mucus or slime. With continuing diarrhoea he has lost weight (5 kg in 6 months), despite a good appetite.

Examination

There is evidence of recent weight loss and a mild effusion of the right knee. Otherwise systems examination is normal.

Questions

- What is the differential diagnosis?
- How would you investigate and manage this patient?

ANSWER 81

The combination of diarrhoea and arthritis is not uncommon, and the likeliest diagnoses are either a reactive or enteropathic (i.e. inflammatory bowel disease-associated) arthritis. However, the diarrhoea is too longstanding to consider reactive disease, and inflammatory bowel disease would be likely to cause passage of blood or mucus and other extra-intestinal features such as rashes, ulcers or ocular disease. This history is typical for a malabsorption picture with steatorrhoea leading to fatty foul-smelling stools that float and are hard to flush. This combination of malabsorption and arthritis should make one consider Whipple's disease – and this case is a classical presentation.

Whipple's disease is a systemic illness caused by the Gram-positive bacillus *Tropheryma whippelii*. Due to the multisystem nature of the condition, there is often considerable diagnostic delay and the disease may be quite advanced before correct treatment is instituted. The symptoms of Whipple's disease can be remembered thus:

Weight loss	Diarrhoea
Hyperpigmentation of the skin	Interstitial nephritis
Intestinal pain	Skin rashes
Pleuritis	Eye disease
Pneumonitis	Arthropathy
Lymphadenopathy	Subcutaneous nodules
Encephalopathy (dementia)	Endocarditis
Steatorrhoea	

The arthritis may appear as a migratory seronegative oligo- or polyarthritis, similar to a spondyloarthropathy (there is an association with HLA-B27) and may precede the development of other symptoms by up to 10 years. Synovial fluid from these patients is fairly non-specific and inflammatory, but synovial biopsies may demonstrate the presence of PAS-positive granules in so-called 'foamy' macrophages.

The diagnosis is made either histologically or by PCR. Jejunal biopsy may demonstrate the infiltration of macrophages with diastase-resistant inclusions with positive PAS staining, whereas PCR can be performed on tissue from affected sites such as small bowel, lymph node, synovial tissue and fluid. PCR from peripheral blood does not have a high diagnostic yield.

As for all patients with a malabsorptive history, the investigations should also assess nutritional status, and calcium, B12/iron/folate and vitamin D levels should be checked.

The treatment of Whipple's disease is protracted antibiotic therapy. Seek advice from an experienced infectious diseases unit before commencing therapy.

KEY POINTS
• Although rare, consider Whipple's disease in any patient presenting with malabsorption, weight loss and arthritis.
• The diagnostic test is jejunal biopsy.

CASE 82: CHRONIC EXTENSIVE MUSCLE PAIN

History

A 46-year-old woman is referred to the rheumatology department with a long history of muscle pain and fatigue. Her symptoms developed insidiously and she now complains of pain 'all over her body', poor sleep and exhaustion much of the time. She denies constitutional upset or specific symptoms but is finding it hard to work or care for her family. Her medical history is unremarkable and she takes no regular medications.

Examination

This woman is well and has no peripheral stigmata of inflammatory disease. Although her joints are mildly tender, there is no evidence of synovial thickening or effusion. Palpation of a number of soft-tissue points is tender but her muscle strength is preserved. All systems examinations are normal.

INVESTIGATIONS		
		Normal range
Haemoglobin	14.9 g/dl	13.3–17.7 g/dL
White cell count	8.3×10^9/L	$3.9–10.6 \times 10^9$/L
Platelets	345×10^9/L	$150–440 \times 10^9$/L
Urea	5.8 mmol/L	2.5–6.7 mmol/L
Creatinine	82 µmol/L	70–120 µmol/L
Calcium	2.4 mmol/L	2.12–2.65 mmol/L
Creatine kinase	156 iU/L	25–195 iU/L
Thyroid stimulating hormone	1.2 mU/L	0.3–6.0 mU/L
ESR	8 mm/h	<10 mm/h
CRP	<5 mg/L	<5 mg/L
RF	Negative	
ANA	Negative	

Questions

- What is the likely diagnosis?
- What further investigations are required?
- How would you manage this patient?

ANSWER 82

This patient has chronic pain, fatigue and soft-tissue tenderness in the absence of clinical or serological evidence of inflammatory disease. The likely diagnosis is fibromyalgia, a non-inflammatory syndrome of unknown aetiology. Characteristic features of this condition are diffuse pain, non-restorative sleep and trigger points of hyperalgesia (pain amplification). The symptoms tend to be chronic and are often present for months before patients seek medical advice. In addition to these 'classic' symptoms, patients may complain of arthralgia, morning stiffness, depression, paraesthesiae and even Raynaud's phenomenon.

The diagnostic clinical finding in fibromyalgia (whether primary or secondary) is the presence of trigger points: at least 11 out of a potential 18 specific tender points of hyperalgesia on the surface anatomy. These regions are exquisitely tender to mild pressure (i.e. enough to blanch a thumbnail). The nine pairs of trigger points are:

- occiput: muscle insertions at the base of the skull
- trapezius: midpoint of the muscle belly
- supraspinatus: medial border of scapula spine
- gluteal: upper outer quadrant
- greater trochanter: posterior to greater tronchanter
- low cervical: muscle belly anterior to C5–7 spaces
- second rib: second costochondral junction
- lateral epicondyle: 2 cm distal to epicondyles
- knee: proximal to medial joint line.

Since the differential diagnosis of fibromyalgia encompasses inflammatory joint and connective tissue diseases, a limited screening set of investigations is appropriate, but the difficulty is deciding when to stop. The batch of investigations listed above effectively rules out the most common diagnoses and therefore this patient does not require further tests. Although primary fibromyalgia is non-inflammatory and therefore associated with normal investigations, secondary fibromyalgia is not uncommon in patients with inflammatory disease such as rheumatoid arthritis or SLE. In these cases, abnormal clinical findings and laboratory results reflect the primary inflammatory disorder, rather than fibromyalgia per se.

The management of fibromyalgia has many components. Patient reassurance on several points is crucial.

- Fibromyalgia is a real disease and they are not 'mad' or 'making it up'.
- Although disabling, fibromyalgia is not destructive or a threat to long-term health.
- Although many of the symptoms can be treated pharmacologically, self-management is very effective and they have considerable control over the condition.

A combination of patient reassurance, education, graded aerobic exercise and management of sleep disturbance can be very successful. The most common pharmacological intervention (which covers many of the components of treatment listed above) is a low-dose tricyclic antidepressant such as amitriptyline; if side-effects such as dry mouth or drowsiness cause problems, selective serotonin reuptake inhibitors may prove beneficial.

 KEY POINTS

- Fibromyalgia is a non-inflammatory syndrome characterized by chronic pain, poor sleep and low mood.
- It commonly coexists with inflammatory disease such as RA or SLE.
- Patient reassurance is a critical component of therapy.

CASE 83: INTRACTABLE SYNOVITIS

History

A 54-year-old woman is reviewed in the rheumatology clinic. She was diagnosed with seropositive rheumatoid arthritis 14 years ago with prolonged early-morning stiffness, a small-joint arthropathy and a marked acute-phase response (elevated ESR and C-reactive protein). Despite aggressive therapy with disease-modifying agents, she has never achieved disease remission, continues to struggle with joint pains and stiffness and struggles with activities of daily living. Her livelihood is at risk as she is unable to type effectively. She has previously tried methotrexate but it produced marked nausea and deranged liver function tests at 15 mg/week and had to be stopped. Hydroxychloroquine and azathioprine were both ineffective. Current medications are leflunomide 20 mg once-daily, prednisolone 4 mg once-daily, alendronate 70 mg weekly and calcichew D3 forte once-daily.

Examination

This woman has marked synovitis with tenderness and swelling of many of her metacarpophalangeal (MCP) and proximal interphalangeal (PIP) joints, her right wrist and left knee. A radiograph is shown in Fig. 83.1.

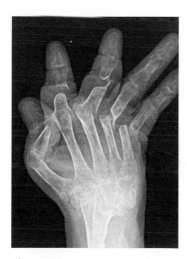

Figure 83.1

INVESTIGATIONS		
		Normal range
ESR	67 mm/h	<10 mm/h
CRP	97 mg/L	<5 mg/L

Questions
- How is disease activity formally measured in rheumatoid arthritis?
- What form of therapy is available to this patient?
- What are the associated risks of that type of treatment?

ANSWER 83

This woman has severe rheumatoid arthritis (RA) that is refractory to standard DMARD therapy, her current treatment being leflunomide, a pyrimidine synthesis inhibitor, and low-dose prednisolone. Her hand and wrist X-ray reveals advanced destructive rheumatoid disease, with extensive erosions, bone loss and joint destruction.

Disease activity in RA is measured by the disease activity score (DAS), which is a composite score of the clinical evidence of synovitis, the current inflammatory response and the patient's own assessment of their health. Clinical synovitis is scored by counting the number of tender and swollen joints out of a total of 28 (shoulders, elbows, wrists, MCPs, PIPs and knees). The patient's 'global health' is determined by using a visual analogue score system: the patient is presented with a horizontal line 100 mm long with 0 (no arthritis activity) at one end and 100 (severe arthritis activity) at the other and is asked to mark where on the line she feels her overall health lies. This is measured with a ruler and expressed out of 100. A DAS calculator (available on-line) is required to calculate the DAS and levels of activity are recorded as high (>5.1), moderate (3.2–5.1), low (2.6–3.19) and remission (<2.6). This patient would certainly have a high disease activity score.

Patients who have high disease activity as determined by the DAS and have either failed or failed to tolerate standard disease modifying therapy qualify for biologic therapy – monoclonal antibodies that are directed against key components of the inflammatory response.

The first-line biologic therapy in use currently is with anti-TNF-α (such as infliximab or adalimumab, both monoclonal antibodies directed against TNF-α, or etanercept, a fusion protein that acts as a decoy receptor for TNF-α). TNF-α blockade is highly effective in up to 70 per cent of patients, reducing both inflammation and the progressive structural damage associated with severe active disease. All TNF inhibitors work best if co-prescribed with methotrexate, even at low doses, but a few are licensed as monotherapy. Although generally safe and well-tolerated, the greatest risk is of increased infection rates. Of particular concern is the reactivation of latent tuberculosis, so screening with a chest X-ray is mandatory before commencing treatment. As TNF-α is also a 'tumour surveillance' molecule, there is a theoretical risk of increased malignancy with this treatment. This has not been borne out in long-term safety data, with the possible exception of lymphoma. However, the association between anti-TNF and lymphoma is also confounded by the fact that patients with severe RA are more likely to develop lymphoma, regardless of anti-TNF exposure.

Second-line biologic therapies for RA include:

- rituximab – a monoclonal antibody directed against CD20-positive B-cells, and commonly used for those who fail to respond to TNF blockade
- abatacept – a decoy receptor preventing T-cell co-stimulation and activation
- tocilizumab – a monoclonal antibody directed against the IL-6 receptor.

Patients on biologic therapy should be carefully monitored and assessed for adequate clinical response by rheumatology units with experience in the use of these agents.

KEY POINTS

- Patients with active RA despite DMARD therapy may qualify for biologic therapy.
- TNF-α inhibition is the first-line biologic therapy.
- All patients should be screened for tuberculosis prior to commencing treatment.

CASE 84: HAEMOPTYSIS AND RENAL FAILURE

History
A 58-year-old woman is admitted to the emergency department with haemoptysis. She has been non-specifically unwell with recurrent low-grade fever, non-productive cough and weight loss for the last few weeks but is now 'exhausted' and short of breath on exertion. Her general practitioner had done some blood tests and commenced oral antibiotics with no benefit and she has been coughing up blood for 24 hours. Her medical history includes type 2 diabetes for which she takes metformin. She is a smoker with a 20-pack per year history and is teetotal.

Examination
This woman looks unwell and sounds nasally congested. She is not febrile. Pulse rate is 88/min, blood pressure 145/92 mmHg and oxygen saturations 95 per cent on room air. There are fine inspiratory crackles in the mid and lower zones of the chest, but cardiovascular and abdominal examination is unremarkable. A radiograph is shown in Fig. 84.1.

🔎 INVESTIGATIONS

		Normal range
Haemoglobin	10.9 g/dL	13.3–17.7 g/dL
Mean corpuscular volume (MCV)	85 fL	80–99 fL
White cell count	7.4×10^9/L	$3.9–10.6 \times 10^9$/L
Platelets	523×10^9/L	$150–440 \times 10^9$/L
ESR	62 mm/h	<10 mm/h
CRP	94 mg/L	<5 mg/L
Urea	28.4 mmol/L	2.5–6.7 mmol/L
Creatinine	312 µmol/L	70–120 µmol/L
cANCA	Strongly positive	
Anti-PR3	Strongly positive	

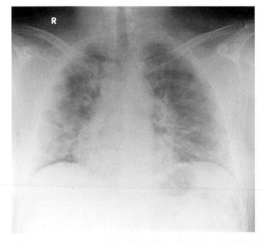

Figure 84.1

Questions
- What is the differential diagnosis?
- Is there a gold standard diagnostic investigation?
- How would you treat this patient?

ANSWER 84

Although one should consider malignancy in any smoker presenting with haemoptysis and an abnormal chest X-ray, the rapid renal impairment, constitutional upset and marked inflammatory response make it more likely to be an inflammatory pulmonary–renal syndrome such as a vasculitis, systemic lupus erythematosus (SLE) or Goodpasture's disease. In addition, the chest X-ray is typical of pulmonary haemorrhage rather than malignancy, with diffuse alveolar infiltrates and a 'bat's wing' appearance of perihilar shadowing. The presence of cANCA (cytoplasmic antineutrophil antibody) and anti-PR3 (antiproteinase) antibody suggest Wegener's granulomatosis, although neither is diagnostic and both may be raised in malignancy or other vasculitides.

The gold standard investigation would be a tissue biopsy to identify the presence of a granulomatous vasculitis. This patient with a raised creatinine would certainly require a renal biopsy for both diagnostic and prognostic purposes.

The classic triad of Wegener's granulomatosis is the presence of upper and lower respiratory tract disease and renal impairment.

!	Clinical features of Wegener's granulomatosis	
Upper airway	Sinuses and nasal mucosa	Chronic sinusitis Nasal discharge and crusting Epistaxis Perforation of nasal septum (saddle-nose deformity)
	Oro-pharyngeal mucosa	Mouth ulcers Suppurative otitis media
	Laryngeal mucosa	Subglottic stenosis Hoarseness and stridor
Lower airway	Chronic inflammation	Cough Nodules (often cavitating) Fixed infiltrates
	Capillaritis	Alveolar haemorrhage Fleeting infiltrates
	Pleuritis	Pleural effusion
Renal disease	Focal, segmental, necrotizing glomerulonephritis	Haematuria and proteinuria Renal impairment Hypertension
Skin		Palpable purpura Nodules
Musculoskeletal		Arthralgia Myalgia
Neurological	Peripheral Central	Mononeuritis multiplex Cerebrovascular events Seizures Diffuse white matter disease

The treatment for Wegener's granulomatosis depends on the severity and extent of organ involvement. 'Limited' Wegener's affects only the upper respiratory tract and low-dose septrin (oral trimethoprim/sulfamethoxazole) may prove beneficial. Oral steroids are of value in more severe disease and the steroid-sparing agent methotrexate may be used (with caution in combination with septrin). Deterioration of renal function and/or pulmonary haemorrhage carry significant mortality and are indications for high-dose intravenous steroids, cyclophosphamide and/or plasma exchange.

 KEY POINTS

- Small-vessel vasculitis may cause a pulmonary–renal syndrome.
- Wegener's granulomatosis is characterized by upper and lower airway disease and renal involvement.
- Nasal crusting, epistaxis and hearing loss are crucial symptoms to identify in the history of a patient with suspected Wegener's granulomatosis.

CASE 85: DIARRHOEA AND A SWOLLEN KNEE

History

A 28-year-old man presents to the emergency department with an acutely painful and swollen right knee. The symptoms began 24 hours previously and have not responded to non-steroidal anti-inflammatory drugs (NSAIDs). He denies fever or constitutional upset. His medical history is unremarkable, except for a self-limiting but severe diarrhoeal illness 3 weeks previously.

Examination

This young man appears well but uncomfortable. His right eye has an injected sclera and there is a moderate effusion in his right knee which is warm and displays reduced range of movement. He has a pustular rash on both heels. The remainder of the examination is normal.

INVESTIGATIONS		
		Normal range
Haemoglobin	16.2 g/dL	13.3–17.7 g/dL
White cell count	9.3×10^9/L	3.9–10.6×10^9/L
Platelets	542×10^9/L	150–440×10^9/L
ESR	45 mm/h	<10 mm/h
CRP	63 mg/L	<5 mg/L

Questions
- What is the differential diagnosis, and which diagnosis is most likely?
- How would you manage this patient?

ANSWER 85

The differential diagnosis in this case of acute monoarthropathy includes:

- acute septic arthritis
- reactive arthritis
- enteropathic arthritis (i.e. associated with inflammatory bowel disease)
- psoriatic arthritis
- gonococcal arthritis
- ankylosing spondylitis
- crystal arthropathy (gout or pseudogout)
- Behçet's syndrome.

Although this patient is systemically well and septic arthritis is therefore relatively unlikely, it should always be included in the differential as its consequences are so dire. The presence of altered bowel habit makes reactive arthritis and enteric arthritis likely contenders; the rash might suggest psoriatic arthritis; but the combination of rash, ocular disease, self-limiting diarrhoea and an acute monoarthropathy make reactive arthritis the most likely diagnosis.

Reactive arthritis is an inflammatory mono- or oligo-arthritis that occurs 1–4 weeks after extra-articular infection, particularly by organisms with a predilection for mucosae (classically genitourinary or gastrointestinal). The most frequently implicated organisms are *Chlamydia* (NB asymptomatic in women), *Salmonella*, *Shigella*, *Yersinia* and *Campylobacter*. Reactive arthritis is the most common inflammatory arthritis affecting young adult men and, in addition to the arthropathy, may cause an enthesopathy or a dactylitis; patients who are HLA-B27-positive are at greater risk of protracted oligo-articular disease and spinal or sacroiliac involvement. Reactive arthritis is associated with a number of extra-articular features which should be specifically sought in the history of anyone presenting with an acute mono-or oligo-arthropathy.

! Extra-articular features of reactive arthritis	
Constitutional	Low-grade fever
Ocular	Conjunctivitis Anterior uveitis
Gastrointestinal	Infectious colitis Sterile colitis
Cutaneous	Circinate balanitis (painless ulceration on glans) Keratoderma blennorrhagica (pustular rash on palms and soles) Erythema nodosum Hyperkeratotic nails
Genitourinary	Infectious urethritis and discharge Sterile urethritis and discharge Prostatitis Vulvovaginitis and salpingitis
Mucosal	Painless oral ulcers

Reiter's syndrome (as originally described) is considered a form of reactive arthritis with a triad of urethritis, conjunctivitis and arthritis following infectious diarrhoea. Not all patients with reactive arthritis have all components of the triad, and the term is best avoided.

The patient in this case has typical investigation results, with non-specific evidence of inflammatory disease. There is no diagnostic test for reactive arthritis, but diagnosis is based on a combination of the clinical picture and cultures from swabs, urine and stool. Synovial fluid cultures are, of course, negative. HLA-B27 is more prevalent in patients with reactive arthritis than the normal population and may help with prognostication, but it is not of value diagnostically. Radiographs are only helpful in chronic disease, when sacroiliitis, ankylosis, enthesopathy, osteopenia and erosion may be evident.

Reactive arthritis is generally benign, with up to 80 per cent making a full recovery. In anticipation of this, first-line treatment for the arthritis is NSAIDs and/or localized therapy in the form of aspiration and injection of the affected joint(s) with corticosteroid and local anaesthetic. This would be an entirely appropriate approach in this case. For those patients with refractory disease, disease-modifying agents such as methotrexate or sulphasalazine are generally effective. The mucocutaneous features of reactive arthritis are usually mild and self-limiting and may not require specific treatment. Liaison with ophthalmological services for management of ocular disease is prudent, particularly in cases of anterior uveitis. In cases with a clearly identified antecedent organism, antibiotic therapy should also be commenced; this is particularly crucial for *Chlamydia* infection in women, which may lead to reduced fertility in the future.

 KEY POINTS

- Consider reactive arthritis in any patient presenting with a monoarthropathy.
- HLA-B27 is useful prognostically but not diagnostically in reactive arthritis.

CASE 86: SWOLLEN ANKLES AND A RASH

History

A 28-year-old African-American man presents to the rheumatology department with a 2-week history of painful swollen ankles and a rash over his shins. His rash is fluctuating with crops of raised tender lumps that fade spontaneously. His ankle pain initially responded to a non-steroidal anti-inflammatory drug (NSAID), but over the last few days has deteriorated such that he finds it hard to walk. His medical history is unremarkable, except for an acutely painful red eye several months previously for which he saw an ophthalmologist and was given steroid eye-drops. He cannot recall the diagnosis he was given at the time. Systems review is unremarkable.

Examination

This man has synovitis affecting both ankles, with a mild effusion on the left and lesions suggestive of resolving erythema nodosum over his shins.

Questions

- What is the likely diagnosis?
- What investigations would be helpful?
- How would you treat this patient?

ANSWER 86

The likely diagnosis is sarcoidosis. Sarcoidosis or sarcoid is a multisystem inflammatory disorder characterized by the presence of non-caseating granulomas in affected organs (commonly lungs, skin, eyes and joints). The presence of ankle disease and erythema nodosum is classic and when associated with bilateral hilar lymphadenopathy is referred to as Löfgren's syndrome. Although of acute onset, this has a more benign outlook than chronic disease as it is exquisitely responsive to steroid therapy.

! Features of sarcoidosis	
Pulmonary	Hilar lymphadenopathy and infiltrates
	Upper airway disease (sinusitis, laryngeal inflammation)
Arthropathy	Classically ankles
	Also knees, wrists and proximal phalangeal joints (PIPs)
	Dactylitis if chronic
Ocular disease	Anterior and/or posterior uveitis
	Keratoconjunctivitis
	Proptosis
Cutaneous disease	Erythema nodosum
	Subcutaneous lesions and lupus pernio if chronic
Parotid enlargement	Xerostomia
Neurological	Mononeuritis multiplex
	Facial nerve palsy
Cardiac	Conduction problems
	Cardiomyopathy

The most important investigation in this case is a chest X-ray to rule out pulmonary involvement. Sarcoidosis is staged according to the development of pulmonary infiltrates and a restrictive pattern on spirometry:

- Stage 0: Normal
- Stage 1: Bilateral hilar lymphadenopathy
- Stage 2: Bilateral hilar lymphadenopathy and pulmonary infiltrates
- Stage 3: Pulmonary infiltrates and restrictive lung disease.

Destructive bony lesions are characteristically absent in sarcoidosis unless the disease is chronic. Where present, they are most commonly found in the hands, with soft-tissue swelling, osteopenia, erosions and periosteal reactions. The wrists and metacarpophalangeal (MCP) joints are generally spared in sarcoid, which may help to differentiate sarcoid from erosive disease such as rheumatoid. Although an elevated angiotensin-converting enzyme (ACE) level is frequently requested in cases of suspected sarcoidosis, it has little diagnostic value as many with acute sarcoid have a normal ACE level and it is frequently elevated in other conditions. The serum calcium must be measured; it may be elevated as granulomas may enhance production of 1,25-dihydrocholecalciferol. Overall, the diagnosis of sarcoidosis is usually clinical/radiological, but can be confirmed by the detection of non-caseating granulomas on biopsy (e.g. lung, lymph node).

Treatment of sarcoidosis depends on the severity and the extent of organ involvement. In this case, his relatively mild arthritis and skin disease may respond to NSAIDs, colchicine or low-dose corticosteroid. Higher doses may be required for persistent arthritis (and methotrexate as a steroid-sparing agent may be beneficial in these cases). If one joint is particularly troublesome, an intra-articular injection of steroid may abort an acute attack. Ocular disease may also respond to topical steroid therapy, as it did in this patient. More powerful systemic immunosuppression such as cyclophosphamide is reserved for neurological or life-threatening disease.

KEY POINTS

- Consider sarcoidosis in any patient presenting with ankle synovitis.
- All patients with sarcoid arthropathy should have a chest X-ray to identify potential respiratory involvement.

CASE 87: RASH, TESTICULAR PAIN AND ARTHRALGIA

History

A 63-year-old man presents to his general practitioner with painful hands. His hands have been stiff and sore for several months but he denies frank swelling. The arthralgia is associated with a 'blotchy rash' over his trunk, profound fatigue and weight loss. In addition, he has experienced bouts of testicular pain and over the last 48 hours has developed central abdominal pain after each meal.

Examination

This man has evidence of recent weight loss and a blue/purple net-like rash over his abdomen and thighs. His joints are tender but there is no clinical evidence of synovitis. Genitourinary examination is unremarkable and he has mild abdominal tenderness to deep palpation but no organomegaly. The remainder of the examination is unremarkable.

INVESTIGATIONS		
		Normal range
Haemoglobin	11.9 g/dL	13.3–17.7 g/dL
Mean corpuscular volume (MCV)	85 fL	80–99 fL
White cell count	7.4×10^9/L	$3.9–10.6 \times 10^9$/L
Platelets	482×10^9/L	$150–440 \times 10^9$/L
ESR	82 mm/h	<10 mm/h
CRP	94 mg/L	<5 mg/L
Rheumatoid factor	Negative	
Anti-CCP antibody	Negative	
Anti-nuclear factor	Negative	
Anti-neutrophil cytoplasmic antibody	Negative	

Questions

- What is the likely diagnosis?
- What test(s) might help confirm the diagnosis?
- How would you manage this patient?

ANSWER 87

The symptom that causes most concern in this case is abdominal pain after eating: such postprandial symptoms raise the suspicion of mesenteric ischaemia. The rash over his abdomen and thighs is characteristic of livedo reticularis, and the patient's marked inflammatory response is somewhat out of keeping with his otherwise relatively mild clinical presentation. The possibility of vasculitis must therefore be considered in this case. Vasculitis can also cause marked constitutional upset and a normocytic anaemia and thrombocytosis, all of which are evident in this patient. The symptom that points to a particular diagnosis is testicular pain, which occurs most frequently in polyarteritis nodosa.

Polyarteritis nodosa is an uncommon vasculitis of small and medium-sized arteries which leads to a varied presentation. The most common features are listed in the box.

! **Clinical features of polyarteritis nodosa**

- Constitutional: malaise, fever, weight loss
- Cutaneous: palpable purpura, ulceration, livedo reticularis
- Musculoskeletal: myalgia, arthralgia, arthritis
- Renal: glomerulonephritis, leading to hypertension
- Gastrointestinal: mesenteric angina
- Neurological: mononeuritis multiplex, stroke, seizures
- Genitourinary: testicular pain

The diagnosis of polyarteritis nodosa can be difficult as there are no diagnostic serological markers and the autoimmune profile is characteristically negative. There is an association with hepatitis B and hepatitis serology should be checked in all patients with suspected vasculitis. Once the diagnosis is suspected, a tissue diagnosis should be sought from a biopsy of an affected organ (e.g. skin, testicle, sural nerve). Angiography is the investigation of choice if biopsy is not possible – and is crucial in this case to investigate/delineate mesenteric arteritis. Typical findings of mesenteric arteriography in polyarteritis nodosa are small aneurysms, occlusions and stenoses.

The treatment of polyarteritis nodosa depends on the extent and severity of the disease, but steroids, steroid-sparing agents and cyclophosphamide are all used commonly; this patient would certainly require high-dose steroids and cyclophosphamide to prevent intestinal ischaemia and infarction. Plasmapheresis and antiviral therapy are recommended as alternative treatment for patients who are positive for hepatitis B.

 KEY POINTS

- Consider mesenteric ischaemia in any patient presenting with a systemic illness and postprandial abdominal pain.
- Testicular pain is a characteristic feature of polyarteritis nodosa.
- Polyarteritis nodosa has an association with hepatitis B infection.

CASE 88: PAINFUL HANDS AND DRY EYES

History

A 44-year-old woman presents to the rheumatology department with a long history of sore, stiff hands and dry, painful eyes. She delayed seeking medical attention as she was concerned she had developed rheumatoid arthritis. The pain in her hands affects principally her wrists, metacarpophalangeal (MCP) and proximal interphalangeal (PIP) joints with protracted early-morning stiffness. Her eyes feel 'gritty' much of the time, getting worse as the day progresses such that they are very painful by the end of the day. During her worst symptoms she complains of photophobia. She has recently noticed a reduction in saliva and finds it difficult to eat dry foods without 'washing them down with water'. Her medical history is unremarkable and she is on no regular medication.

Examination

This woman is well with mild synovitis of her wrist, MCPs and PIPs. Her sclerae are minimally injected but there is no discharge and her acuity is normal. The remainder of her examination is normal.

INVESTIGATIONS		
		Normal range
Haemoglobin	11.1 g/dL	13.3–17.7 g/dL
Mean corpuscular volume (MCV)	85 fL	80–99 fL
White cell count	8.3×10^9/L	$3.9–10.6 \times 10^9$/L
Platelets	432×10^9/L	$150–440 \times 10^9$/L
ESR	45 mm/h	<10 mm/h
Rheumatoid factor	35 iU/mL	<11 iU/mL
Anti-nuclear factor	Positive 1:640	
Anti-Ro antibody	Detected	
Anti-La antibody	Detected	
Immunoglobulins	Polyclonal hypergammaglobulinaemia	

Questions
- What is the diagnosis?
- What test gives an objective indication of dry eyes?
- How would you manage this patient?
- What complication may arise from her condition?

ANSWER 88

The combination of dry eyes, dry mouth and an inflammatory arthritis is highly suggestive of Sjögren's syndrome. Sjögren's syndrome may occur as a primary condition (associated with anti-nuclear antibodies to Ro and La) or in association with another connective tissue disease, most commonly RA. The exocrine glands become destroyed by a lymphocytic infiltration which impairs tear and saliva production; the arthritis mimics the distribution of RA but tends to be milder and non-erosive.

The most common symptoms of Sjögren's syndrome are:

- dry eyes and dry mouth (xerostomia)
- arthritis
- parotid gland enlargement
- Raynaud's phenomenon
- constitutional upset (fever, fatigue)
- rashes (cutaneous vasculitis, photosensitivity)
- dyspareunia.

The objective assessment of dry eyes is based on the Schirmer's test. A standardized piece of filter paper is hooked under the lower eyelid and the amount of paper-wetting over 5 minutes is measured. Less than 5 mm would be highly suggestive of decreased tear production.

The overall prognosis of Sjögren's syndrome is generally more benign than that of other inflammatory diseases. Treatment of this patient would be essentially symptomatic.

Dry eyes may be improved by wearing spectacles with side shields to reduce evaporation; eye-drops (preservative-free artificial tears or lacrilube ointment) are required in many patients. For those with severe disease, ophthalmology services may offer punctal occlusion to reduce tear drainage. Severe surface disease such as scleritis or ulcers may need topical steroids. Xerostomia may respond well to sugar-free sweets to stimulate saliva production. All patients must pay particular attention to dental hygiene as accelerated caries is a frequent problem. For those with disabling lack of saliva production, cholinergic drugs such as pilocarpine may be helpful but are associated with muscarinic side-effects such as sweating or gastrointestinal disturbance. Her arthritis will probably respond promptly to non-steroidal anti-inflammatory drugs (NSAIDs), hydroxychloroquine or low-dose prednisolone.

Sjögren's syndrome is often associated with a polyclonal hypergammaglobulinaemia and may progress to the development of a lymphoma. The risk of this transformation is probably less than originally estimated and may be less than 10 per cent. However, many units would still screen with annual immunoglobulin profiling and patients should be vigilant about the development/progression of lymphadenopathy or parotid swelling. Although not relevant in this case, anti-Ro and anti-La antibodies cross the placenta and cross-react with the developing conducting system in the fetal heart. As a result, patients of child-bearing age with Ro and La antibodies should be counselled regarding potential fetal heart-block and should have antenatal care through an experienced high-risk obstetric unit.

 KEY POINTS

- Dry eyes and a dry mouth are common symptoms in Sjögren's syndrome.
- Sjögren's syndrome is associated with anti-Ro and anti-La antibodies.
- Patients with anti-Ro or anti-La antibodies who are pregnant should be reviewed by a high-risk obstetric unit as there is risk of heart block in the developing fetus.

CASE 89: GENITAL ULCERS AND A RASH

History

A 26-year-old Turkish man presents to his general practitioner with a painful apthous ulcer on his scrotum. Although he has had oral ulcers on and off 'for years', this is the first episode in the genitourinary tract. He denies other genitourinary symptoms and is not sexually active. Four weeks previously he experienced a rash over the front of his shins: discrete red tender lumps appeared and then faded spontaneously, going through colour changes like a bruise. On systems review he mentions that his right knee is intermittently painful and swollen, but denies any other problems.

Examination

This young man has a deep ulcer on his scrotum, but his penis is normal. He has no oral ulcers. The sclera of his right eye is injected. He has a solitary brown slightly raised lesion on his left shin and a small effusion in the right knee. He has an erythematous lesion in the left antecubital fossa from blood donation 48 hours previously.

Questions
- What diagnosis does this patient's combination of symptoms suggest?
- What is your differential diagnosis?
- What other features would you seek in the history?
- Is his racial origin relevant?
- What are the treatment options?

ANSWER 89

The combination of orogenital ulceration, arthritis, conjunctivitis and a rash suggests a diagnosis of Behçet's syndrome. The rash is a classic description of erythema nodosum, a panniculitis associated with a number of inflammatory conditions; the skin reaction to needlestick (in this case venesection for blood donation) is an example of pathergy, which may be pathognomonic of Behçet's disease.

Behçet's is an autoimmune disease that affects men and women equally. However, this patient's racial origin is certainly helpful in this case as Behçet's is more common in those from Turkey, the Mediterranean and the Far East. The geographical risk is probably a function of the disease's association with HLA-B51. Although there are a number of specific features which are typical of Behçet's disease (outlined below), many are shared with other inflammatory conditions and Behçet's can present a diagnostic challenge.

! Symptoms and signs of Behçet's disease	
Recurrent oral ulceration	At least three attacks per year
Recurrent genital ulceration	Most common on scrotum or vulva Prone to scarring
Ocular disease	Anterior or posterior uveitis Conjunctivitis Corneal ulceration
Cutaneous disease	Erythema nodosum Pathergy Pseudofolliculitis/papulopustular lesions
Arthritis	Classically migratory mono- or oligoarthritis
Vascular diseases	Thrombosis and arterial aneurysms
Neurological disease	Headache Aseptic meningoencephalitis Intracranial hypertension may be due to venous sinus thrombosis

The differential diagnosis for ulceration, arthritis, ocular disease and a rash is broad. You must consider:

- Crohn's disease
- reactive arthritis
- systemic lupus erythematosus
- vasculitis
- sarcoidosis (although ulceration is atypical).

Owing to the breadth of the differential diagnosis, a detailed history and examination (looking for specific features of the above) is mandatory. Unfortunately there is no diagnostic test for Behçet's disease and laboratory findings are non-specific with an elevated acute-phase response and a polyclonal hypergammaglobulinaemia.

The treatment of Behçet's depends on the constellation and severity of the symptoms. Mucocutaneous disease can be effectively treated with colchicine, dapsone or thalidomide. In more severe disease, steroids (± steroid-sparing agents) or tacrolimus may be required. Cyclophosphamide is generally reserved for life- or sight-threatening disease.

KEY POINTS

- Although rare, consider Behçet's syndrome in patients presenting with orogenital ulceration and arthritis.
- The presence of the pathergy reaction may be helpful in the diagnosis of Behçet's syndrome.

CASE 90: RASH, ARTHRALGIA AND FACIAL WEAKNESS

History

A 32-year-old American woman presents with flu-like symptoms, painful hands and loss of power down the right side of her face. She was previously fit and well but on a recent trip back to Wisconsin sustained an insect bite to the back of her knee and started to feel unwell a week later. Her main complaints at that stage were headaches and fatigue, with arthralgia in her hands, all of which she self-managed with paracetamol and non-steroidal anti-inflammatories until her return to the UK. A few weeks have elapsed, but she woke this morning with unilateral weakness of her facial muscles, including the forehead.

Examination

This woman has a large (15 cm) circular rash over the back of her knee with a bright red border and central clearing. Although her joints are tender, she has no clinical evidence of synovitis. She has a facial nerve palsy on the left side.

Questions

- What is the diagnosis?
- List its potential complications.
- What test would you order?
- How would you manage this patient?

ANSWER 90

The combination of rash leading to arthralgia and cranial neuropathy is a classic presentation of Lyme disease. It is a multisystem disease caused by infection with the tick-borne spirochaete *Borrelia burgdorferi*; the *Ixodes* tick commonly lives on deer and is endemic in parts of the United States (including Wisconsin, as in this case). Lyme disease has three clinical stages.

- Stage 1 is localized cutaneous disease. Classic sites for the tick to bite are warm, moist areas like the back of the knee, axillae and under the breast. However, the tick is very small and only half of patients with clear-cut Lyme disease may remember the bite. The characteristic rash, called erythema chronicum migrans, develops from the bite, first as a macule and then a spreading annular lesion with central clearing. This stage is associated with constitutional upset; fever and lymphadenopathy are not uncommon. Arthralgia, rather than arthritis, is also a feature. Stage 1 tends to last a few weeks.
- Stage 2 is disseminated disease. It characteristically occurs within a few months of the rash and is dominated by neurological syndromes. The most common presentations are cranial neuropathies (particularly the seventh cranial nerve, as in this case), headaches, meningoencephalitis and mononeuritis multiplex. Cardiac manifestations include heart block and myocarditis. Although arthralgia and peri-articular disease are not uncommon, true synovitis occurs only in stage 3 disease.
- Stage 3 produces chronic infection up to two years after the initial infection and leads to asymmetrical oligoarthritis, particularly at the knee.

Diagnosis of Lyme disease is based on the clinical picture and serological evidence of antibodies to *Borrelia*, but test results are complicated by a high rate of false positives in endemic areas and false negatives in early disease. The prompt use of antibiotics in stage 1 may also diminish diagnostic yield. PCR, however, can detect *Borrelia* DNA in blood, synovial fluid and tissue and cerebrospinal fluid.

The treatment of Lyme disease is antibiotic therapy, the dose and route of administration depending on stage and severity of disease. Second- and third-generation cephalosporins tend to be the treatment of choice, with oral courses of up to 1 month for cutaneous disease alone and intravenous regimens for disseminated disease, but expert advice should be sought from microbiological services. Localized joint disease may respond well to intra-articular injection, synovectomy or hydroxychloroquine in addition to antimicrobial therapy.

 KEY POINTS

- Lyme disease occurs following a tick bite.
- The characteristic features are rash, arthritis and nerve block.
- Treatment is with antimicrobial therapy.

CASE 91: RASH AND ABDOMINAL PAIN IN AN ADOLESCENT

History
A 17-year-old youth is referred urgently to the rheumatology department with a rapidly progressing rash over his buttocks and legs, and severe, cramping abdominal pain. The rash began as flat, red areas which became 'bumpy' and then developed into palpable dark red–purple lumps that fail to blanch on pressure. The abdominal pain occurs in spasms and does not appear to relate to food. His bowel habit is unchanged.

Examination
This youth is well but clearly very uncomfortable. His pulse rate is 84/min and blood pressure 117/62 mmHg. He has palpable purpura over his buttocks and the backs of his legs. His right ankle is mildly synovitic but otherwise his joints are normal and he has no other stigmata of inflammatory disease. Palpation of his abdomen reveals diffuse tenderness but no guarding or rebound. There is no organomegaly and normal bowel sounds are audible.

🔍 | INVESTIGATIONS

A urine dipstick reveals 3+ protein but no blood.

Questions
- What are the common causes of purpura?
- What is the likely diagnosis in this case?
- How can this diagnosis be confirmed?
- How would you manage this patient?

ANSWER 91

Purpura are the result of a spontaneous extravasation of blood from the capillaries into the skin. If small they are known as petechiae, when they are large they are termed ecchymoses. There is an extensive differential diagnosis for purpura:

! Causes of purpura	
Infection	Meningococcal disease (consider in any patient as it carries a high mortality) Infective endocarditis Septicaemia
Thrombocytopenia	Idiopathic thrombocytopenic purpura Thrombotic thrombocytopenic purpura Marrow failure of any cause
Vascular defect	Senile or steroid-induced purpura Vasculitis (especially Henoch–Schönlein purpura)
Coagulation defect	Haemophilia
Drugs	Steroids Sulphonamides

The combination of palpable purpura (distributed particularly over the buttocks and extensor surfaces of legs), abdominal pain, arthritis and renal disease is a classic presentation of Henoch–Schönlein purpura (HSP). HSP is a distinct and frequently self-limiting small-vessel vasculitis that can affect any age; but the majority of cases present in children aged 2–10 years, in whom the prognosis is more benign than the adult form, often remitting entirely within 3–4 months. The abdominal pain may mimic a surgical abdomen and can presage intussusception, haemorrhage or perforation. The arthritis, in contrast, is relatively mild and tends to affect the knees and ankles. Renal disease is generally mild in children, but its presence and severity determine the prognosis of the condition. Many will experience only a mild glomerulitis with microscopic haematuria, but a crescentic glomerulonephritis may occur, with the development of nephrotic syndrome or acute renal failure.

The diagnostic test is a skin biopsy which reveals a leucocytoclastic vasculitis with IgA deposition in the affected blood vessels; IgA is also detectable in the renal mesangium.

Treatment depends on the severity of the disease. In mild cases, no specific therapy is necessary. The arthritis will in general respond to non-steroidal anti-inflammatory drugs (NSAIDs); steroid therapy is reserved for those with severe abdominal symptoms. If renal disease is severe (deteriorating renal function, hypertension, nephrotic syndrome or crescents on renal biopsy), high-dose steroids and cytotoxics such as cyclophosphamide may be effective first-line; plasma exchange or intravenous immunoglobulin may be tried in refractory cases.

KEY POINTS

- Consider HSP in a patient with purpura affecting the back of the legs preferentially.
- Abdominal pain in these patients is a sinister symptom.
- The disease is milder in children and frequently remits spontaneously.

CASE 92: WEIGHT LOSS AND CLAUDICATION IN A YOUNG WOMAN

History

A 24-year-old Asian woman presents to her general practitioner with dramatic weight loss and intermittent fever. Her symptoms have been present for several weeks, but over the last few days she has developed difficulty walking. Although previously very fit and active, she can now walk only a quarter of a mile before developing fatigue and cramping pain in her calves that forces her to stop. Once she has rested for a while, she is able to continue walking again, but the symptoms return.

Examination

This young woman is well but her GP is unable to detect a blood pressure from the left arm: the pulses are absent on that side and a subclavian bruit is clearly audible. The opposite arm is normal. Further examination of her vascular system reveals another bruit over her right femoral artery with decreased pulses distally on the same side. The rest of her pulses are present and the remainder of her physical examination is normal.

Questions

- What is the likely diagnosis?
- Are any particular blood tests helpful prior to referral?
- What investigation will the rheumatology department request?
- What is the management of this condition?

ANSWER 92

This patient gives an excellent history of claudication. She has both symptoms and signs of vascular insufficiency but is far too young to have straightforward atheromatous disease. The most likely cause is a large-vessel vasculitis and her age and racial origin make Takayasu's arteritis the most likely cause.

Takayasu's arteritis is an occlusive vasculitis leading to stenoses of the aorta and its principal branches. The symptoms and signs of the disease depend on the distribution of the affected vessel but upper limbs are generally affected more commonly than the iliac tributaries. There are three phases to the disease:

- initial pre-pulseless stage with constitutional upset (fever, weight loss)
- inflammatory stage with vessel pain and tenderness
- pulseless stage with ischaemic symptoms.

Since the disease is a chronic relapsing and remitting condition, patients do not proceed predictably through individual stages but may experience all three types of symptoms simultaneously.

There are no specific blood tests for suspected Takayasu's arteritis, but the detection of an elevated inflammatory response and an anaemia of chronic disease or thrombocytosis are supportive, so a full blood count and ESR might prove useful at the point of referral. The investigation of choice that the rheumatology department will request is angiography, which reveals long-segment stenoses. Although MR angiography (MRA) is an alternative and carries no radiation risk, it may miss more proximal or distal stenoses. If the clinical picture and arteriography are characteristic, there is no need to proceed to biopsy.

The mainstay of treatment is high-dose corticosteroids plus a steroid-sparing agent such as methotrexate. Bone protection is mandatory with the corticosteroids, and aspirin and antihypertensives should also be considered. Cyclophosphamide is reserved for those patients who do not achieve remission with standard therapy. Surgical intervention such as bypass or angioplasty may improve ischaemic symptoms once the inflammation is under control.

 KEY POINTS

- Takayasu's arteritis is known as the pulseless disease and is a cause of vascular insufficiency in those too young for atheromatous disease.
- Angiography is diagnostic.
- Surgery may be required once the patient is in remission.

CASE 93: SWOLLEN CHEEKS IN AN ELDERLY MAN

History

A 79-year-old man presents to his general practitioner with bilaterally swollen cheeks. He also complains of feeling 'tired all the time', weight loss and occasional night sweats. Although he admits to an irritating dry cough he denies frank breathlessness or change in exercise tolerance. His medical history includes hypertension, for which he takes ramipril.

Examination

This elderly man is slightly pale, with bilateral parotid enlargement and cervical lymphadenopathy.

Questions

- What is the differential diagnosis for bilateral parotid enlargement?
- What other symptoms would you ask about in the history?
- What would you look for on physical examination?
- What screening tests would you consider?
- What is the most likely diagnosis in this case?

ANSWER 93

The most common causes for bilateral parotid swelling in adults include:

- Sjögren's syndrome
- sarcoidosis
- lymphoma.

This patient's symptoms are relatively non-specific but there are some direct questions that may lead you to suspect one potential diagnosis over another.

Patients with Sjögren's syndrome may report dry eyes (often described as gritty rather than dry) or a dry mouth, complaining that biscuits and bread are particularly difficult to swallow without water. Arthralgia is also a feature, but may be present in the other conditions too. Dry eyes are assessed using Schirmer's test: if the patient demonstrates appropriate wetting of filter paper placed under the lower eyelid, significant Sjögren's is unlikely. Screening tests for Sjögren's include rheumatoid factor, ANA and anti-Ro and anti-La antibodies.

Sarcoidosis tends to present with ankle (peri)arthritis, erythema nodosum and respiratory symptoms due to interstitial lung disease. Lymphadenopathy and hepatosplenomegaly may also be evident on examination. Screening tests for sarcoidosis include checking calcium and angiotensin-converting enzyme (ACE) levels and a chest X-ray.

Lymphoma is one of the great mimics in medicine and can present in a myriad of ways. The classic symptoms are of night sweats and weight loss; examination findings may be limited to lymphadenopathy and hepatosplenomegaly. Investigations include immuno-globulins and serum electrophoresis.

This man has no history of the most common sicca features evident in Sjögren's or the arthropathy or rash associated with sarcoid. Although his dry cough might make you consider sarcoid-related lung disease, his exercise capacity is undiminished and the ACE inhibitor ramipril is the more likely culprit. His relatively advanced age makes malignancy one of the more likely differentials, and the combination of weight loss, night sweats, parotid swelling and lymphadenopathy makes lymphoma the most likely diagnosis in this case.

 KEY POINTS

- Bilateral parotid enlargement may be due to Sjögren's syndrome, sarcoidosis or lymphoma.
- Presentations of all three conditions may be relatively non-specific and rely on direct questioning.
- Simple specific investigations may help to differentiate between potential causes.

CASE 94: A SWOLLEN KNEE

History

A 35-year-old woman is seen in the emergency department with an acutely swollen left knee. Despite the swelling, she complains of only minimal pain in the knee. There is no history of trauma and she is otherwise entirely well with no other joint problems. She denies risk factors for inflammatory disease and is on no regular medication.

Examination

Beyond a slightly warm effusion of the left knee her examination is totally unremarkable. The admitting senior house officer aspirates the effusion and discovers haemorrhagic synovial fluid.

Questions
- What is the differential diagnosis?
- Which is the most likely in this case?
- How would you confirm the diagnosis?
- How would you manage this patient?

ANSWER 94

This woman has a haemarthrosis. The most common causes of blood in the joint are:

- trauma
- bleeding diathesis (including over-anticoagulation)
- connective tissue disease (e.g. Ehlers–Danlos syndrome)
- synovial tumours.

Given that she is previously fit and well, with no history of trauma and no features of connective tissue disease, the discovery of haemorrhagic synovial fluid should raise the possibility of a synovial tumour.

The most common primary synovial tumour is pigmented villonodular synovitis (PVNS). PVNS is a benign tumour of the synovium or tendon sheath (in which case it is called giant cell tumour of tendon sheath) which presents with isolated swelling in or near an isolated joint or tendon. The tumour may invade into surrounding bone, causing erosions or cysts.

The diagnosis is generally confirmed by arthroscopy, biopsy and histological examination. Macroscopically the synovium is pigmented and prolific with multiple villi, fronds and nodularity. The histology is characteristic with demonstration of histiocytes, haemosiderin-containing cells and multinucleated giant cells. Alternatively (and probably most appropriate in this case), MRI is also diagnostic as it highlights the haemosiderin-laden nodules.

Management of PVNS is surgical, with complete synovectomy via an arthroscopic approach.

 KEY POINTS

- Consider synovial tumours in a patient with unexplained haemarthrosis.
- MRI is generally diagnostic.

CASE 95: A CHILD WITH A SWOLLEN KNEE

History

A six-year-old girl is brought to her general practitioner by her mother, with an 8-week history of a stiff and painful swollen right knee. There is no recall of trauma and she is otherwise well, with no recent history of infective illness. Her medical history is unremarkable and her vaccinations are all up to date. A course of a non-steroidal anti-inflammatory drug (NSAID) has been of minimal benefit.

Examination

The girl is uncomfortable getting undressed and on to the examination couch. There are no peripheral stigmata of inflammatory disease, but she has a moderate effusion of the right knee, which is warm and shows reduced flexion.

INVESTIGATIONS		
		Normal range
Haemoglobin	14.9 g/dL	13.3–17.7 g/dL
White cell count	$7.4 \times 10^9/l$	$3.9–10.6 \times 10^9/L$
Platelets	$423 \times 10^9/L$	$150–440 \times 10^9/L$
ESR	22 mm/h	<10 mm/h
C-reactive protein	34 mg/L	<5 mg/L
Rheumatoid factor	Negative	
Anti-nuclear factor	Positive	

Questions

- What is the likely diagnosis?
- How is this arthritis classified?
- What is the relevance of the positive ANA?
- How would you manage her?

ANSWER 95

This young girl has a persistent inflammatory arthopathy and an elevated acute-phase response, which makes the likely diagnosis juvenile idiopathic arthritis (JIA). JIA affects up to 0.1 per cent of the population and is classified broadly into:

- oligoarticular arthritis (<5 joints; subdivided into persistent and extended)
- polyarticular arthritis (>5 joints; subdivided into RF positive and RF negative)
- systemic-onset JIA
- enthesitis-related arthritis
- psoriatic arthritis
- other (not meeting above criteria).

The most common presentation for JIA is oligoarticular disease and (as in this case) the knee is most commonly affected. Although initially fewer than five joints are affected, after 6 months of disease the arthritis may progress to affect more than five joints; this so-called 'extended oligoarthritis' carries a worse prognosis than the persistent counter-part. It is critical to bear in mind that up to 20 per cent of children with oligoarticular disease develop anterior uveitis and the risk is higher in children who are ANA positive, so this form of immunological screening is advisable. Since anterior uveitis may be asymptomatic, early referral to ophthalmology services for slit-lamp examination is also appropriate. If present, treatment of anterior uveitis is with topical steroid.

Polyarticular JIA essentially mirrors adult rheumatoid arthritis, with the exception of two features: (a) the majority of polyarticular JIA patients are RF negative, and (b) JIA may affect the distal interphalangeal joints (although curiously not in those who are RF positive!). Systemic JIA disease has an identical presentation to adult-onset Stills with spiking fevers, a salmon-pink evanescent rash, lymphadenopathy, hepatosplenomegaly and inflammatory arthritis. Enthesitis-related arthritis is linked to the presence of HLA-B27 and often affects the lower limb, most commonly the foot, and sacroiliitis is rarer than in adult disease. Childhood psoriatic arthritis tends to present as an oligoarthritis.

Fortunately children are generally more resistant to drug toxicity from NSAIDs or disease-modifying antirheumatic drugs (DMARDs). Given that this patient has not improved on NSAIDs, it would be appropriate to opt for an intra-articular injection of steroid into the affected knee and then resort to methotrexate in the face of recurrent problems. For children with severe or resistant disease, the biologic therapy of choice is etanercept, although it may cause flares of eye disease in a minority of cases.

 KEY POINTS

- The most common presentation of juvenile idiopathic arthritis is oligoarticular disease.
- Check ANA status in a child with inflammatory oligoarthritis as it highlights those at greater risk of developing anterior uveitis.
- Children tolerate NSAIDs and DMARDs better than adults!

CASE 96: ACNE, ARTHRALGIA AND CHEST PAINS

History
A 22-year-old woman consults her general practitioner complaining of fever, joint pains and chest pain. The joint pains began 3 weeks previously and affect the small joints of her hands and wrists with moderate early-morning stiffness. The muscle pains are relatively non-specific and are not associated with any loss of power. Overall she has derived some benefit from treatment with regular non-steroidal anti-inflammatory drugs (NSAIDs). In the last 48 hours, however, she has also developed a low-grade fever and a sharp right-sided chest pain on deep inspiration. She denies breathlessness or cough and has no risk factors for pulmonary embolus. Her medical history includes acne, for which she has been taking minocycline for the past year.

Examination
This young woman is well, with a normal respiratory rate and oxygen saturations. Her temperature is 37.6°C. Although her joints are tender she has no objective evidence of synovitis. Respiratory examination reveals a pleural rub over the painful area in the right lower zone anteriorly but is otherwise normal.

The GP was concerned she has developed systemic lupus erythematosus (SLE) and ordered some basic blood tests and an immunology screen.

🔍 INVESTIGATIONS		
		Normal range
Haemoglobin	13.2 g/dL	13.3–17.7 g/dL
White cell count	7.6 × 10⁹/L	3.9–10.6 × 10⁹/L
Platelets	326 × 10⁹/L	150–440 × 10⁹/L
ESR	4 mm/h	<10 mm/h
C-reactive protein	2 mg/L	<5 mg/l
Creatine kinase	74 iU/L	25–195 iU/L
Rheumatoid factor	Negative	
ANA	Positive 1/320	
Anti-histone antibody	Positive	

Questions
- What is the possible diagnosis?
- How would you manage this patient?

ANSWER 96

This young woman has presented with arthralgia, serositis, a low-grade fever and positive anti-nuclear and histone antibodies. Her full blood count, inflammatory markers and CK are normal, mitigating against infection, rheumatoid arthritis, SLE or inflammatory myopathy. The use of the tetracycline minocycline for acne makes drug-induced lupus the most likely unifying diagnosis.

Drug-induced lupus (DIL) generates a different spectrum of clinical manifestations from idiopathic disease. DIL is less severe than idiopathic SLE, and nephritis or central nervous system involvement is very rare. This case highlights the classic manifestations of DIL with fever, myalgias, arthralgia/arthritis and pleuritis all being apparent. Interestingly a significant proportion of DIL patients with pulmonary involvement develop infiltrates, which is relatively uncommon in idiopathic disease. In addition, the malar and discoid rashes that are so characteristic for SLE are less common in DIL.

The diagnosis of DIL is made on the basis of the clinical picture, the presence of a precipitating drug and the immune profile, which may help to differentiate drug-induced and idiopathic disease.

! **Immunological profiles of SLE and DIL**		
Autoantibody	*Idiopathic SLE*	*Drug-induced lupus*
Anti-nuclear antibody (ANA)	Positive	Positive
Anti-histone antibody	Common	Very common
dsDNA antibody	Common	Rare
Anti-Sm, anti-Ro, anti-La	Common	Rare, if ever
Hypocomplementaemia	Frequent	Rare

The most common drugs responsible for a lupus-like syndrome are procainamide, hydralazine, quinidine, isoniazid, methyldopa, chlorpromazine and minocycline. Interestingly minocycline induces anti-histone antibodies only in up to 15 per cent of cases, and up to three-quarters of patients generate a positive pANCA.

Treatment involves stopping the offending medication and the symptoms will gradually resolve. Some patients may use a course of NSAIDs to tide them over and a very small minority with severe symptoms (e.g. pleuritis) may require corticosteroids.

It is worth remembering that the positive ANA may persist for months or even years after resolution of the symptoms and it is not clinically relevant. Re-challenge with the precipitating drug should be avoided wherever possible.

KEY POINTS
• Drug-induced lupus is less severe than SLE.
• It is generally associated with anti-histone antibodies.
• Clinical manifestations will disappear on stopping the drug, but the ANA may persist for months or years.

CASE 97: A BREATHLESS PATIENT WITH LUPUS

History

A 38-year-old man with an earlier diagnosis of systemic lupus erythematosus (SLE) is admitted to the emergency department with progressive breathlessness. His diagnosis was made several years previously while resident in India, on the basis of rashes, arthralgia, ulcers and 'lots of bad antibodies'. He was prescribed medication but admits he has never complied except for a brief period when he took warfarin. He has become progressively more breathless over the last few months, with his exercise tolerance falling from unlimited to only a few metres. He admits that his lupus symptoms have also been deteriorating over the same period. There is no history of cough or infective symptoms.

Examination

This man has a marked malar rash and is short of breath at rest (18 breaths per minute). His oxygen saturations on room air are 92 per cent at rest and on minimal exercise drop to 85 per cent. His pulse rate is 93/min, blood pressure 118/68 mmHg. His jugular venous pulse (JVP) is elevated with systolic v waves, and he has a pansystolic murmur over the tricuspid area. There is also pulsatile hepatomegaly and pitting oedema to his knees. Examination of the respiratory system is unremarkable.

Questions

- What is the differential diagnosis for the patient's breathlessness?
- How would you investigate him?
- What are the treatment options?

ANSWER 97

This patient has progressive breathlessness, desaturates on exercise and has features of right heart failure and tricuspid regurgitation. The diagnosis is pulmonary arterial hypertension (PAH). The three main causes of PAH in patients with lupus include:

- interstitial lung disease
- pulmonary vasculopathy
- chronic thromboembolism.

In this case, vasculopathy or chronic pulmonary embolisms are the most likely given the absence of clinical features of interstitial lung disease and his prior history of warfarinization.

! Appropriate investigations for PAH	
Arterial blood gas	Assessment of respiratory failure
Pulmonary function tests	Identification of restrictive lung disease Evaluation of gas transfer as measure of disease severity
Chest X-ray	Evidence of interstitial lung disease Peripheral 'pruning' of vascular tree in occlusive vascular disease
Echocardiography	Characterize degree of tricuspid regurgitation Estimation of pulmonary arterial pressure Evaluation of right ventricular function
CT-PA	Investigation of chronic thromboembolic disease
HRCT	Evaluation of interstitial lung disease (inflammatory vs fibrotic change)
Cardiac catheterization	Formal evaluation of right heart pressures Assessment of reversibility with vasodilators

In addition, the patient should have a full assessment for the complications of his SLE, including an antibody and anti-phospholipid profile. His peripheral oedema is probably due to right heart failure; and his blood pressure is normal, suggesting his renal system is uninvolved, but nonetheless his urine should be checked for protein and/or casts.

Management of PAH in these circumstances is based on management of the resultant right heart failure with diuretics, digoxin to improve ventricular contractility and lifelong anticoagulation. Patients who demonstrate improvement in their pulmonary pressures with vasodilators may benefit from calcium-channel blockade, intravenous prostacyclin analogues or the endothelin antagonist bosentan. These patients should be referred to specialist cardiorespiratory units experienced in the management of pulmonary arterial hypertension.

 KEY POINTS

- Pulmonary hypertension may develop as a complication of SLE.
- Basic investigations to assess the severity of PAH include chest X-ray, pulmonary function tests and echocardiography and CT.
- Any patient with evidence of PAH should be referred promptly to a specialist unit for further management.

CASE 98: ANAEMIA AND WEIGHT LOSS IN A PATIENT WITH RHEUMATOID ARTHRITIS

History

A 79-year-old woman with longstanding rheumatoid arthritis (RA) is reviewed in clinic. Despite methotrexate therapy she has some persistent but mild early-morning stiffness and swelling affecting her hands and wrists. She complains of being exhausted all of the time and with a reduced appetite, and she has lost several kilograms in weight in the last two months. She is a non-smoker and drinks only occasionally. Apart from the methotrexate she takes only paracetamol for pain. There is no other relevant medical histroy and review of systems is otherwise normal.

Examination

This elderly woman is pale with evidence of recent weight loss. She has minimal synovitis in her metacarpophalangeal (MCP) joints and wrists. Examination is otherwise unremarkable.

INVESTIGATIONS		
		Normal range
Haemoglobin	8.2 g/dL	13.3–17.7 g/dL
Mean cell volume	78.2 fL	83–105 fL
White cell count	9.3 × 10⁹/L	3.9–10.6 × 10⁹/L
Platelets	242 × 10⁹/L	150–440 × 10⁹/L
ESR	21 mm/h	<10 mm/h
C-reactive protein	24 mg/L	<5 mg/L

Questions

- What are possible causes of weight loss in a patient with rheumatoid arthritis?
- What is the most likely cause in this case?
- What is the most important investigation?

ANSWER 98

Weight loss is common in patients with inflammatory disease. The most important diagnoses to consider are:

- disease activity (likely, due to high levels of circulating cytokines, including TNF-α)
- occult infection
- malignancy.

In this case, the patient undoubtedly has uncontrolled disease activity; but her symptoms and dramatic weight loss are out of keeping with her mild synovitis and only moderate inflammatory response, so one should keep an open mind as to the underlying cause.

The critical feature of her full blood count is that the patient is profoundly anaemic. Rheumatoid arthritis may case anaemia in several ways:

- anaemia of chronic disease
- drug-induced due to disease-modifying agents, such as methotrexate
- iron deficiency due to gastrointestinal blood loss (consider NSAID-induced peptic ulcer disease or malignancy)
- associated haemolytic anaemia.

The majority of these causes lead to either normocytic or macrocytic anaemia; this patient has microcytic red cells which suggest iron deficiency. Her reduced MCV is even more marked considering her methotrexate therapy, which normally leads to a macrocytosis. Bear in mind that patients may develop anaemia for reasons independent of their underlying inflammatory disease, so it is unwise to attribute a new anaemia simply to their rheumatoid arthritis. A common cause of iron-deficiency anaemia in this age-group is gastrointestinal malignancy, and this patient's associated weight loss is also highly suggestive of an occult cancer. The investigation of choice in this case is endoscopy of the upper and lower gastrointestinal tracts to identify a bleeding source, either an ulcer or tumour.

 KEY POINTS

- Anaemia and weight loss are both common in inflammatory disease and may be a reflection of disease activity.
- Keep an open mind as to the underlying diagnosis in the presence of new clinical features, or symptoms and signs that are out of keeping with the level of disease activity.
- The important other diagnoses to consider are occult infection or malignancy.

CASE 99: A BREATHLESS PATIENT WITH DERMATOMYOSITIS

History
A 45-year-old woman has been admitted to the rheumatology ward with a diagnosis of dermatomyositis. She is profoundly weak (muscle power 2/5 in all proximal groups) and on admission received a pulse of intravenous methylprednisolone and cyclophosphamide. She remains on 60 mg prednisolone orally, bone protection and thromboprophylaxis. Ten days after admission her muscle strength has not improved and the senior house officer is asked to review her as she has become acutely more breathless.

Examination
This woman appears exhausted and unwell with marked peripheral myopathy. She has a temperature of 37.8°C and her oxygen saturation is 88 per cent on room air. Her pulse rate is 92/min and blood pressure 125/86 mmHg. Her jugular venous pulse (JVP) is not elevated and her heart sounds are normal with no peripheral oedema or evidence of deep venous thrombosis. She is short of breath at rest (20 breaths per minute) with reduced chest wall movements bilaterally. Her right mid-zone is dull to percussion with increased vocal resonance. There are mild crackles throughout which clear with coughing.

Questions
- What is the differential diagnosis of breathlessness in this patient?
- What are the appropriate investigations?
- How would you manage her?

ANSWER 99

Patients with severe muscle weakness have several reasons for breathlessness. The main differential diagnoses to consider are:

- ventilatory failure due to respiratory muscle weakness
- pneumonia, including due to aspiration and particularly in those who have received immunosuppression
- interstitial lung disease
- pulmonary embolus due to immobility.

The clinical features in this case (fever and findings consistent with pneumonia), on a background of profound immunosuppression, would make pneumonia the most likely explanation for her deterioration. Infection is a significant problem in this patient population: respiratory muscle weakness may lead to atelectasis and collapse which increase the risk of infection. In addition, her orophayngeal muscles may be involved, leading to aspiration. Although interstitial lung disease occurs in 5–10 per cent of dermatomyositis patients, it typically develops more insidiously and presents with late or pan-inspiratory crackles that do not clear with coughing (such clearing would be more suggestive of transmitted sounds from upper airway secretions). Although she is on thromboprophylaxis which reduces the chance of pulmonary embolus and there is no history of pleuritic chest pain or haemoptysis and her JVP is normal, thromboembolism should always be considered.

Appropriate immediate investigations include:

- arterial blood gas to assess respiratory failure
- blood cultures to assess for infection
- chest X-ray looking for features of bronchopneumonia, collapse or interstitial lung disease
- spirometry to assess reduction in vital capacity.

It would be appropriate to commence broad-spectrum antibiotics intravenously to cover for aspiration and nosocomial infection (advice should be sought from local microbiology services). She should receive chest physiotherapy to help clear secretions and reduce the risk of lobar collapse. These patients may deteriorate rapidly and early review by respiratory and intensive care teams is appropriate.

 KEY POINTS

- The differential diagnosis of breathlessness in patients with dermatomyositis includes infection, ventilatory failure, interstitial lung disease and thromboembolism.
- Chest physiotherapy is central to management and should be instituted early.
- Seek advice from respiratory and intensive care teams promptly.

CASE 100: ASTHMA, RHINITIS, FOOT DROP AND A RASH

History

A 45-year-old woman presents to the emergency department unable to lift her right foot. She was well the night before and noticed the problem immediately on waking in the morning; she came straight to hospital as she was frightened she was having a stroke. Her past medical history reveals poorly controlled adult-onset asthma for which she takes inhaled steroids and beta-agonist, and persistent rhinitis for which she uses nasal spray. She has no cardiovascular risk factors. She takes no oral medication and has no other relevant medical or family history. Her only foreign travel was a two-week holiday in Menorca 4 years ago. She does not smoke or drink.

Examination

This woman is well and not febrile. She walks with a high-stepping gait on the right side to avoid her toes dragging on the floor. She has weakness of dorsiflexion and eversion of the foot, with some reduced sensation over the top of the foot. There is a non-blanching rash over her legs which she reports has been present for a week and is gradually deteriorating. The remainder of her examination is normal.

INVESTIGATIONS		
		Normal range
Haemoglobin	14.2 g/dL	13.3–17.7 g/dL
White cell count	9.3×10^9/L	$3.9–10.6 \times 10^9$/L
Neutrophils	5.0×10^9/L	$2.0–7.0 \times 10^9$/L
Eosinophils	1.3×10^9/L	$0.0–0.5 \times 10^9$/L
Platelets	242×10^9/L	$150–440 \times 10^9$/L
ESR	45 mm/h	<10 mm/h
C-reactive protein	69 mg/L	<5 mg/L
Urea	5.2 mmol/L	2.5–6.7 mmol/L
Creatinine	92 μmol/L	70–120 μmol/L

Questions
- What is the likely diagnosis?
- What are the other major clinical features of the underlying condition?
- How would you confirm the diagnosis?
- What treatment is recommended?

ANSWER 100

This patient has the clinical features of an acute common peroneal nerve palsy, with foot drop and loss of sensation over the dorsum of the foot. In the absence of traumatic nerve injury, the most likely underlying cause is mononeuritis multiplex. The most common causes of mononeuritis multiplex are diabetes mellitus and the vasculitides; she has no history of diabetes but does present with a vasculitic rash, history of adult-onset asthma, rhinitis and a marked peripheral eosinophilia. The unifying diagnosis that encompasses all these features is Churg–Strauss syndrome.

Churg–Strauss syndrome is a granulomatous vasculitis of small and medium-sized vessels in association with a peripheral eosinophilia. It usually presents in those with a history of allergy and the major clinical features listed in the box.

❗ Major clinical features of Churg–Strauss syndrome	
System	*Clinical features*
Sinuses	Rhinitis (up to 75%), sinus pain and tenderness
	Nasal polyps
Respiratory	Adult-onset asthma
	Pulmonary infiltrates (shifting and patchy)
Neurological	Mononeuritis multiplex
	Symmetrical polyneuropathy
Cardiovascular	Pericardial effusion
	Cardiomyopathy
Dermatological	Petechiae, purpura and infarction
	Subcutaneous nodules
Gastrointestinal	Pain
	Bloody diarrhoea
Musculoskeletal	Arthralgias

The diagnosis should be considered in any patient presenting with evidence of vasculitis (in this case, non-blanching rash and mononeuritis multiplex), history of adult-onset asthma, rhinitis or nasal polyposis and a peripheral eosinophilia. A significant proportion of patients have antineutrophil cytoplasmic antibodies (characteristically pANCA) and may have an elevated IgE. The diagnosis is often confirmed with biopsy of an affected organ (skin, nerve) which reveals a necrotizing vasculitis and small extravascular granulomas with central eosinophilic cores.

Churg–Strauss disease responds well to corticosteroid therapy. In this case, in which neurological involvement is a predominant feature, high-dose oral prednisolone (1 mg/kg up to 60 mg daily) or a pulse of intravenous methylprednisolone would be appropriate. Bone protection would also be mandatory and consideration may be given to the use of steroid-sparing agents (e.g. methotrexate or azathioprine) if dose reduction proves hard to achieve. Cyclophosphamide treatment is generally reserved for those with life- or organ-threatening disease.

KEY POINTS

- Mononeuritis multiplex is a common presentation of systemic vasculitis.
- Consider Churg–Strauss syndrome in any patient with vasculitis, allergic history and eosinophilia.
- Churg–Strauss syndrome responds well to corticosteroid therapy.

INDEX

References are by case number with relevant page number(s) following in brackets.